CLINICIAN TO EDUCATOR
WHAT EXPERTS KNOW
IN OCCUPATIONAL THERAPY

EDITED BY
KAREN SLADYK, PhD, OTR, FAOTA
BAY PATH COLLEGE
LONGMEADOW, MASSACHUSETTS

SLACK
INCORPORATED

an innovative information, education, and management company

6900 Grove Road • Thorofare, NJ 08086

Publisher: John H. Bond
Editorial Director: Amy E. Drummond
Design Editor: Lauren Biddle Plummer

Published by: SLACK Incorporated
                  6900 Grove Road
                  Thorofare, NJ 08086 USA
                  Telephone: 856-848-1000
                  Fax: 856-853-5991
                  www.slackbooks.com

Printed in the United States of America

Last digit is print number: 10   9   8   7   6   5   4   3   2

CONTENTS

CONTRIBUTING AUTHORS

Alexandra A. Bell, PhD, PT
University of Connecticut
Storrs, CT

Roxie M. Black, MS, OTR/L
University of Southern Maine
Lewiston-Auburn College
Lewiston, ME

Sherry Borcherding, MA, OTR
University of Missouri, Columbia
Columbia, MO

Jeffery L. Boss, MS, OTR
Texas Tech University Health Sciences Center
Lubbock, TX

Nancy Dooley, MA, OTR
New England Institute of Technology
Warwick, RI

Nancy A. Everhardt, MOT, MEd, OTR
Texas Tech University Health Sciences Center
Lubbock, TX

Christina Griffin, MAEd, OTR
Arizona School of Health Sciences
Phoenix, AZ

Anne Birge James, MS, OTR/L
University of Hartford
West Hartford, CT

Marijke Kehrhahn, PhD
University of Connecticut
Storrs, CT

Nancy MacRae, MS, OTR/L, FAOTA
University of New England
Biddeford, ME

Henriette Pranger, PhD
Eastern Connecticut State University
Willimantic, CT

Karen Sladyk, PhD, OTR, FAOTA
Bay Path College
Longmeadow, MA

Lori G. Sladyk, MS, CSE
Rockville High School
Vernon, CT

Brenda Smaga, MS, OTR/L
Bay Path College
Longmeadow, MA

Vicki Smith, MBA, OTR/L
University of Tennessee at Chattanooga
Chattanooga, TN

PREFACE

How lucky I am to be able to combine my love of occupational therapy and adult education in a monograph that is designed for new faculty in occupational therapy. The monograph idea was born when I saw new faculty with no idea where to start, and remembered when I was in the same boat. It is so hard going from a clinician's job where you are an expert to a faculty position where you are a novice. I found mentors and so did my new peers, but I thought, "Wouldn't it be great if someone wrote these things down so new faculty had a place for advice?"

So that's where this monograph begins: a collection of advice to our peers; a place to start with ideas but not pre-scriptions; also, a list of common problems that pop up in academia that are different from the clinical world. All the authors send their best wishes along with their ideas.

As the millennium arrived, invitations were sent to the community of educators electronically and by flyer to invite submissions to the monograph. A variety of topics were suggested and the chapters and briefs included in this monograph only begin to address the possible topics for a new educator. Perhaps we can expand the list in the future.

As the editor, I organized the submitted chapters and briefs in themes. I tried to fill in any gaps with informational briefs I wrote. As you can see by the Table of Contents, the chapters and briefs are very diverse, from simple to complex. Two monograph sections focus on the teaching life and the academic career. The teaching life section provides practical advice on managing the classroom-related activities of faculty. The academic career section focuses on managing the day-to-day career of the educator. Educators looking for further information on an academic career are encouraged to read Robinson's *From Clinician to Academician*, published by the American Occupational Therapy Association.

As with any project, there are many, many people to thank. First, Amy Drummond, my friend, who did not laugh when I told her about this idea and then argued my cause to the people at SLACK Incorporated. To all the great people at SLACK who were willing to try a different idea from what they specialize in. To my sister, who wrote a chapter in her expertise and also kept my feet on the ground by writing little stinging jokes on all my chapters and briefs as she proofread them.

A special thank you to my editorial board of reviewers. Typically, reviewers are experts in the field who volunteer to blindly review and accept papers for publication. In this case, my initial reviewers were expert clinicians but novice educators, having just finished their first year in full-time academia. Who better to read chapters on advice to new educators than new educators? Carol Berry, MS, OTR, and Dyanne Mascia Hanelius, OTR, were excellent reviewers. Lastly, I want to thank the additional blind reviewers who gave feedback on the final draft.

If you are thinking about a career or just starting an academic career, all the authors wish you the best.

Karen Sladyk, PhD, OTR, FAOTA

Section One

MANAGING A
TEACHING LIFE

Chapter One

SUSTAINING THE SPIRIT OF TEACHING

Nancy MacRae, MS, OTR/L, FAOTA, and Roxie M. Black, MS, OTR/L

"Activities of the spirit include any pursuits that nourish the soul by providing opportunities for creating meaning."
—Christiansen, 1997

INTRODUCTION

Becoming an occupational therapy educator is exciting, challenging, and sometimes overwhelming. The occupation of teaching is very different from, and requires skills beyond, that of a clinician. It is easy to get caught up in learning to write syllabi, in good test construction, and in determining what pedagogical approach to adopt and which teaching strategies to explore. And then there are the requirements of scholarship and service!

Beyond the everyday tasks that one must learn to become a good educator and the demands necessary for the job, however, is the need to find what sustains you in this occupation. What makes teaching exciting? What gives the job meaning? Is there a spiritual aspect to the occupation of teaching? The authors of this paper not only believe that the answer to this question is a resounding "Yes!" but have identified how to find and explore the spirit of teaching.

We, the authors of this chapter, graduated from the same Master's of Adult Education program at the University of Southern Maine in 1989. The phrase we each carried with us at that time was the exhortation of our advisor, "Follow your passion!" Those words have become a guiding principle for each of us as we have developed as occupational therapy educators. Eleven years later, that continued passion has led us to directorships of occupational therapy education programs, Nancy at the University of New England and Roxie at the University of Southern Maine, Lewiston-Auburn College. The passion for teaching has evolved into one where we both continue to teach and to model and nurture the process for others.

There are numerous ways to examine the passion for and spirit of teaching. Being pragmatists by nature and pro-fession, we decided to explore the theoretical underpinnings in the field of occupational therapy to try to determine where one finds the spirit or meaning in the occupation of teaching. We wanted to determine where the passion for teaching resides, to share some of what we have learned by teaching those who are beginning their teaching journey, and perhaps most importantly, to ensure that both our own and others' passion for teaching is sustained.

OCCUPATION DEFINED

As we know, humans are occupational beings. We find and make meaning in the things we do—the activities in which we engage. These activities or occupations determine and are determined by our sociocultural roles. Hence, our occupations define us. Our identity is inexorably intertwined with what we do.

A clear and simple definition of occupation is offered by Schkade and Schultz (1992) as "activities characterized by three properties—active participation, meaning to the person, and a product that is the output of a process" (p. 829). Theoretically, occupation has been divided into three performance areas: work, play/leisure, and self-help. Teaching would generally fall into the area of work, although for some of us, the joy and satisfaction we gain from our chosen field makes it sometimes feel more like play. In order to analyze teaching as an occupation and how an individual finds meaning in that occupation, we employed an occupational therapy practice model, the Performance, Environment, Occupation (PEO) Model.

THE MODEL

The PEO Model (Figure 1-1) is one of a number of current models that focuses on occupational performance. It was developed by Christiansen and Baum (1997) to emphasize a view of occupational performance as an interaction between an individual and the environment.

Reprinted from Sladyk, K. (2001). *Clinician to Educator: What Experts Know in Occupational Therapy.* Thorofare, NJ: SLACK Incorporated.

Specifically, it is the transactional process between the person, his or her social and physical environment, and occupation. This model was based on general systems, environmental, neurobehavioral, and psychological theories and addresses society's occupational performance needs. Occupational performance is the result of the transaction between the three components of this model. It is dynamic and requires active involvement, with the expected outcomes of competence and the development of skills.

In order to address occupational performance and to influence successful performance of learners, the "P" in this equation, one needs to know the following: what that individual does in daily life, what motivates him or her, and how the person's characteristics combine with the situation in which occupations are undertaken. Students are engaged in the pursuit of knowledge because of a need. However they may describe that need, they have made a choice to devote time, money, and energy to learn about that which is often a passion for them. Students' occupation at this point is to study. Their occupational performance needs are for learning and the ability to appropriately apply it in relevant environments.

Teachers are the enablers or facilitators (Christiansen & Baum, 1997, p. 62) to help students acquire the skills necessary for the performance of tasks and roles that each learner wishes to fulfill. If educators know the developmental status of their students, they can connect with them on various appropriate levels. Learning about them as individuals will better allow educators to fashion a learning situation that will resonate with them. Additionally, understanding the needs of the learners will help educators develop strategies to better allow them to assimilate the information presented. Finally, understanding the environment in which they will function, with its political and social vagaries and the business orientation of managed care, will help us to better prepare students to be able to effectively practice and/or to be better citizens.

Taking into account each of the three components of this model provides teachers with a holistic picture of students. However, there is something that transpires when all three areas have been directly addressed and when what is being taught connects with the learner. The resulting transaction ideally creates that "just right" challenge, takes advantage of that "teachable" moment, creates that recognition of an insight, that "a-ha!" experience. Not only has the student gained insight but the teacher has been rewarded for aligning all the components at the same time. It is truly a win-win situation, one in which both are ready to enthusiastically continue (to sustain) the journey of discovery. The learners want to apply what they have learned to see whether it will work.

This juncture is not reached magically, although elements of a magical moment do exist. Preliminary work based on learned theory and methodologies and a student-

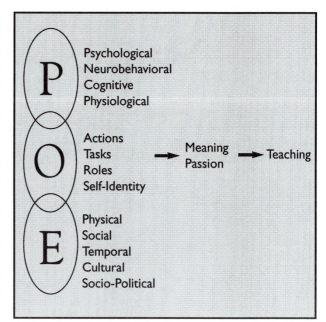

Figure 1-1. POE Model.

centered approach are prerequisites. A plethora of personality characteristics of the teacher such as charisma, empathy, patience, quiet strength, confidence, high expectations, and a sense of humor may add immeasurably to the mix. Some teachers appear to be born to the role, while others need training; yet each is capable of reaching this culminating point if the transactional process is on target. It is a self-fulfilling trait: The student yearns for more such moments; the teacher strives to create such discoveries.

A "WALK THROUGH" THE MODEL

In order to further clarify the model and its use, we will use one of the authors, Roxie Black, as a case study. We will summarize the process and provide examples of how you each may use this approach to evaluate yourself. As we look at the "P" section on the diagram, which is the person who is engaged in the activity, there are various components to examine: the psychological, neurobehavioral, cognitive, and physiological aspects of a person.

Although there are age-related changes in some of these areas for Roxie, middle-age (being in her early 50s in particular) is a wonderful time of life for her. She feels good physically, mentally, and emotionally; has a great zest for life which she shares with her students and colleagues; and has compensated for the mild changes associated with aging that diminishing senses have created. She believes she is a good role model for her students.

The environment component of the model includes the physical, social, temporal, cultural, and sociopolitical world that encompasses the person and either supports or stresses the activities in which a person engages. Roxie's working environment at Lewiston-Auburn College fully supports her teaching activities. The physical and social environment is open, welcoming, and offers a sense of community she has not found elsewhere. Her feminist and multicultural beliefs are encouraged and can flourish in the sociopolitical environment, as can her excitement for teaching and learning.

When examining the final circle in the model that depicts occupation and how it interacts with what we have just discussed, we must examine the task of teaching, considering the actions, tasks, roles, and self-identity inherent in it. Roxie has taught at the college level for 16 years. Over those years, she has learned the importance of establishing a climate of safety in the classroom, where each voice is valued and heard. She teaches in an interactive, student-centered manner, believing that students come to the classroom already having knowledge and will construct their own meaning from information presented based on their previous experiences and knowledge. She ascribes to the tenet outlined by Ira Shor (1992) that education can be empowering. She has high expectations for and expects rigorous work from her students; nevertheless, her classrooms are active, challenging (for both her and the students), and fun.

Roxie sees her role as a facilitator and co-learner in the classroom rather than as the specialist with all the knowledge. She is comfortable and confident in this role and achieves great satisfaction from it. She recognizes herself to be a better than average teacher, and some of the greatest joy she receives from her job occurs in the classroom.

It is the transaction between these three components—the person, the environment, and the occupation—that give meaning to the occupation of teaching. The interaction among Roxie (who she is and what she brings to teaching), the environment where she engages in teaching, and the actual activities of teaching results in that place of excitement and joy, the place where passion resides. When all of these components come together in a perfect manner, a teacher experiences that incomparable joy and excitement that moves her to a spiritual plane. It is the "yesss" experience that moves an educator to strive to reproduce that feeling. Csikszentmihalyi (1990) describes this experience as one of "flow." He views this as the "optimal experience where people enter a state where they are so involved in an activity that nothing else seems to matter" (p. 4). You have been there—when the class seems to fly by, you and the students are totally engaged in learning, and you wonder where the time has gone.

When you as the educator are supported by your environment, using teaching strategies that are meaningful and successful to you and the students, you can achieve this sense of flow, this optimal state of inner experience which many of us view as spiritual in nature, and you can discover the place where passion resides for you. This is what gives meaning to and sustains us in the occupation of teaching.

Spirit/Passion

Attempting to further explain this moment, explorations are needed on both the meaning and the passionate response produced by the transaction. Underlying both meaning and passion is a spiritual dimension. In fact, if we look at the Canadian Model of Occupational Performance (Canadian Association of Occupational Therapists, 1997), spirituality is at its very core. The individual's spirit is deemed to be the individual, the very essential nature of that person, that which the person finds meaningful. Consequently, everything else that the person does will be dynamically affected by his or her spirituality, and what is being done will affect his or her spirituality. Urbanowski and Vargo (1994) have defined spirituality as the "experience of meaning in everyday life" (p. 89). This definition is profound in its simplicity. It allows us to understand that the daily actions of a person and what those daily activities mean to that person are critical. These activities may appear mundane to the observer, but they are not. One has only to work with an individual who has experienced a loss in physical functioning and can no longer perform daily activities to realize how important these daily tasks are to how people feel about themselves.

Passion cannot be viewed separately from meaning, for it is itself imbued with meaning of a great intensity. For an individual to be passionate about something, he or she has ascribed significant value and meaning to it. "Follow your passion" is a freeing charge that contains many emotional facets. What is understood with this statement, though, is an underlying enthusiasm, if not zeal, to pursue that about which one is passionate.

When teaching has meaning for the teacher, the occupational performance (the action) of teaching and seeing the transactional results of teaching in your students is the flame of passion, a passion that is both sated and strengthened at the same time. It validates and increases the desire to do it again and to do it better the next time in a journey of discovery.

This sustaining cycle is fueled by practicing the art and science of teaching and can be tremendously soul-satisfying for the practitioner. We need to attend to these cycles in both the teacher and the learner so that life-long learning is fostered, meaning is exemplified, and passion's embers are reignited and sustained.

If teaching is an occupation of one's choice, it is meaningful. Peloquin (1997) believes that "...meaningful occupation animates and extends the human spirit..." (p.167). That which one finds meaningful is also often a source of passion. Teaching a subject about which one is passionate does resonate beyond the self: It becomes infectious; the learner becomes more interested, if not intrigued; the acquired knowledge is retained better. The feeling and animation that gird the delivery of information are what make it memorable.

Reprinted from Sladyk, K. (2001). *Clinician to Educator: What Experts Know in Occupational Therapy*. Thorofare, NJ: SLACK Incorporated.

Actually being able to teach what one is passionate about is a thrill. To combine the desire to teach with teaching the skills one needs to practice a former and/or concurrent profession is extraordinary. This pairing can often lead to a passionate performance and hopefully inspire/ignite/sustain passion in the learner, thus beginning the renewing cycles previously described.

SUMMARY

Using the PEO Model allows us to identify where the passion resides in the occupation of teaching. A careful analysis of the three components—person, environment, occupation—and their transaction enables teachers to evaluate themselves and the meaning the act of teaching holds for them. If all three of these components are aligned, there can be an ensuing and sustainable passion, what we are calling the meaning and spirit of teaching.

REFERENCES

Canadian Association of Occupational Therapists. (1997). *Canadian Model of Occupational Performance in enabling occupation: An occupational therapy perspective.* Ottawa, Ontario.

Christiansen, C. (1997). Nationally speaking—Acknowledging a spiritual dimension in occupational therapy practice. *American Journal of Occupational Therapy, 51,* 169-172.

Christiansen, C., & Baum, C. (1997). Person-environment occupational performance: A conceptual model for practice. In C. Christiansen & C. Baum (Eds.), *Occupational Therapy: Enabling Function and Well-Being* (2nd ed., pp. 48-70). Thorofare, NJ: SLACK Incorporated.

Csikszentmihalyi, M. (1990). *Flow: The psychology of optimal experience.* New York: Harper Perennial.

Peloquin, S. M. (1997). The spiritual depth of occupation: Making worlds and making lives. *American Journal of Occupational Therapy, 51*(3), 167-168.

Schkade, J., & Schultz, S. (1992). Occupational adaptation: Toward a holistic approach for contemporary practice, part 1. *American Journal of Occupational Therapy, 46*(9), 829-837.

Shor, I. (1992). *Empowering education.* Chicago: University of Chicago Press.

Urbanowski, R., & Vargo, J. (1994). Spirituality, daily practice, and occupational performance model. *Canadian Journal of Occupational Therapy, 61*(2), 88-94.

KNOWING EVERYTHING
Christina Griffin, MAEd, OTR

One thing I have learned in my years of teaching is that you do not have to know everything, even on the subject about which you are lecturing. I no longer feel pressured when asked a question that I have never thought about before or to which I just do not know the answer. For classes in which medical terms are commonly used, I keep a medical dictionary in class and students take turns looking up unfamiliar terms on the spot. This both gives them a chance for self-discovery and helps ensure understanding of the new material to be learned. For more complex questions, I do not assign students to find out the answer because they will soon learn not to ask questions if it causes them more work. I just tell them I do not know, but I will find out and get back to them. I then research the question and give them the answer the very next time I have them in class. I have consistently received positive feedback on student evaluations of teaching for this procedure because students appreciate the prompt feedback and feel that attention has been paid to their individual learning needs. Classes cannot possibly cover every condition or situation that might be encountered in the students' future practice, so this has the added benefit of modeling continuing learning and problem-solving behaviors that students will need to utilize in their clinical practice.

END-OF-CLASS FEEDBACK
Karen Sladyk, PhD, OTR, FAOTA

Each college or university typically has some standard form to be used for class feedback. Unfortunately, some students see this as an opportunity to "get back" at a challenging teacher, or some students are so bored with the forms that they simply check off whatever they feel at the moment (usually under the stress of final exams). Neither feedback provides the instructor with anything meaningful.

Another effective approach is to have students write letters to next year's students telling them how to get the best grade possible in this class. The student should begin the letter with, "In this class I expect to get a (insert grade). To get the best grade possible, I would tell a new student to..."

The letters usually show the correlation between the amount of work the current student applied and grades, a far better measurement than subjective checklists. The educator can adjust class expectations accordingly. For example, if the student wrote that not much is required for an A grade, the faculty may want to raise expectations.

Current students should be told that next year's students will have access to their letters at the beginning of class. Access to the letters helps ground the new students in reality and dispel the myths that may be floating around campus about your class.

Reprinted from Sladyk, K. (2001). *Clinician to Educator: What Experts Know in Occupational Therapy.* Thorofare, NJ: SLACK Incorporated.

Chapter Two

FACILITATING DEVELOPMENT OF STUDENT EXPLICIT AND TACIT KNOWLEDGE

Alexandra A. Bell, PhD, PT

Today you are conducting the first practical exam of the semester for your new class of third-year students. The first student scheduled to take the practical, Susan, did not do well on the first two written exams. Susan tends to speak very little during class meetings. You are pleasantly surprised at her performance in the practical. Though Susan had a slow start, stumbling during her verbal explanation of her choice of treatment for her mock patient, she breezed through the rest of the practical, demonstrating correct evaluation procedures, excellent patient rapport, and adherence to safety protocols.

Mark is the next student scheduled for the practical exam. Mark earned the highest score in the class on the first two written exams. Mark tends to be outspoken and you can depend on him to ask appropriate questions during each class meeting. Mark's performance on the practical is less than satisfactory. Though his verbal explanation of the rationale behind his choice of treatment was accurate and well articulated, his performance was out of sequence, he seemed oblivious to the fact that a person was attached to the hand with which he was working, and he showed little regard for patient safety.

You are perplexed. How could Susan, who has difficulty expressing herself in class, do so well on the practical? How could Mark, who until this exam had the highest GPA in class, earn one of the lowest scores on the practical exam? How can you, the instructor, meet the learning needs of both students?

Occupational therapy students need to be successful in activities that require the acquisition and application of two types of knowledge: explicit knowledge and tacit knowledge. Explicit knowledge is knowledge that is acquired consciously. It is readily retrieved from conscious memory and expressed or explicated in verbal and written formats (Reber, 1993). Knowledge of names and definitions, how things are organized, and simple numerical manipulations are examples of explicit knowledge. Mark, one of the students in the scenario above, demonstrated

accurate explicit knowledge about information covered in the course by earning high grades on the written exams and through his verbal contributions in class.

Tacit knowledge is knowledge one acquires through day-to-day experiences without awareness or intent. It includes knowledge about complex environmental patterns and relationships, contextual cues and consequences, and procedures on how to attain a goal. Tacit knowledge is stored in nonconscious memory. Consequently, tacit knowledge is difficult to articulate or "put into words," yet it is readily put into action (Reber, 1993). Susan, the student, demonstrated appropriate tacit knowledge about treatment procedures and patient interactions in her practical exam performance.

Tacit knowledge is acquired before explicit knowledge (Reber, 1993). For example, students learn the cues that indicate when you will distribute a "pop quiz" in class long before they learn the information they need to pass the quiz. Tacit knowledge is also more "durable" than explicit knowledge. Students may "cram" the names of 20 different microorganisms into memory the night before a pathology exam, yet be able to recall only half those names the following semester. In contrast, most students who learn to perform and practice correct universal precautions procedures are able to apply the procedures in a variety of field training situations without conscious effort.

Age-related differences between explicit and tacit knowledge exist as well. Due to changes in conscious memory functions, the acquisition and application of explicit knowledge tends to decline with age. Tacit knowledge is developed independent of conscious memory. Subsequently, this type of knowledge continues to develop even in the last decades of life (Baltes & Baltes, 1990).

Tacit knowledge appears to be closely linked to one's emotions. Because this knowledge results from experiences of "being in the world," it provides the foundation of knowledge for preferences, biases, and intuitions (Lewicki, 1986; Sheckley & Keeton, 1997). Tacit knowledge is not neces-

Reprinted from Sladyk, K. (2001). *Clinician to Educator: What Experts Know in Occupational Therapy*. Thorofare, NJ: SLACK Incorporated.

sarily accurate. For example, through prior experience, a student may have learned ways of interacting with individuals who have psychiatric impairments that are not appropriate in clinical care contexts. Because this type of knowledge is so durable, "bad habits" are often hard to change.

Though explicit and tacit knowledge are developed differently, the two knowledge bases are not independent of each other. Knowledge gained explicitly, such as complex rules of grammar (e.g., "i before e, except after c"), becomes tacit and "automaticized" after repetition, practice, and application in a variety of contexts (Sternberg, Wagner, Williams, & Horvath, 1995). Conversely, tacit knowledge can be made explicit through conscious efforts to articulate or "talk aloud" as one performs a procedure or reacts to an environmental cue. Through these activities, the tacit knowledge underlying one's actions can be "surfaced" and scrutinized for accuracy and appropriateness (Lewicki, 1986; Sheckley & Keeton, 1997).

Explicit knowledge is gained through learning processes that involve reading, writing, listening, memorizing, and speaking—processes commonly found in the traditional classroom. Tacit knowledge is gained through implicit learning processes. These processes occur as an individual experiences and interacts with his or her environments. Though implicit learning can occur in all environments, instructional settings that tend to enhance implicit learning include laboratory, field training, practicum, and community service. Whereas explicit learning is facilitated when information is presented in a well-organized and sequential manner, implicit learning is facilitated when students are free to observe, explore, and experiment with resources of their own choosing (Sternberg et al., 1995).

For learning to be complete, it must result in the development and utilization of both explicit and tacit knowledge. Without tacit knowledge to guide its application in a variety of contexts, explicit knowledge is reduced to abstract and lifeless information. Students like Mark in the scenario may excel in memorizing and verbalizing "what" and "why" yet be ineffectual in demonstrating "how" and "when." Without explicit knowledge to articulate the reasons behind actions, tacit knowledge becomes a repertoire of automatic behaviors and reactions. Susan was adept in performing procedures in the practical exam, yet unable to explain the rationale behind her performance.

Instructors can meet the learning needs of students, including those like Susan and Mark, by designing and supporting instructional activities that promote both types of knowledge. Consider the following strategies to facilitate the development of student explicit and tacit knowledge.

1. When introducing students to a new domain of knowledge, avoid the temptation to start off with a reading or a lecture, which accentuate the acquisition of explicit knowledge. Rather, engage students first in implicit learning processes in which they can observe domain-related activities, explore elements of the domain in different contexts, and experiment with "how things work" in the domain. Providing first-year students the opportunity to "shadow" experienced clinicians at a clinical site one afternoon a week is an example of an activity that will facilitate the development of tacit knowledge about the profession. Encourage students to link activities to prior experiences and to "use their intuition" to appreciate patterns and relationships among elements of the domain. Do not evaluate student performance at this time. De-emphasize naming, defining, organizing, and memorizing during these activities.

2. Provide opportunities for students to model appropriate patterns of behaviors. Pair up each first-year student with an advanced student who will serve as a "big brother" or "big sister." Support the development of mentor-mentee relationships. Ensure that you, as a member of the faculty, exhibit the behaviors that you want the students to exhibit.

3. To facilitate tacit knowledge development while promoting explicit knowledge acquisition, use graphic concept maps, flow charts, and outlines when first presenting information and during frequent reviews. Provide opportunities for students to make graphic displays of the information they acquire. The graphic displays will help students appreciate patterns and relationships among information components and to recognize gaps in their explicit knowledge base (Sheckley & Keeton, 1997).

4. Support explicit knowledge acquisition by presenting information in a well-organized and sequential manner in an environment that is free from distractions. Whereas tacit knowledge acquisition can take place in complex settings in which relationships are not linear, explicit knowledge acquisition via processes such as reading, writing, and memorizing are hampered in such settings.

5. In the later stages of tacit knowledge acquisition, engage students in activities that help to "bridge the gap" between tacit and explicit knowledge. Activities such as "talk aloud" during the performance of a procedure and reflective writing or reflective dialogue in small groups following an experience can bring to consciousness the tacit knowledge underlying one's actions. Once the knowledge has "surfaced," it can be examined and tested for accuracy, and plans for continued knowledge development can be made (Sheckley & Keeton, 1997).

6. Finally, assess students' knowledge by engaging them in solving ill-defined problems that require the application of both tacit and explicit knowledge to resolve.

Reprinted from Sladyk, K. (2001). *Clinician to Educator: What Experts Know in Occupational Therapy.* Thorofare, NJ: SLACK Incorporated.

Practical exams, like the one in the scenario, that require an integration and demonstration of both types of knowledge to adequately address a clinical case are an excellent method of assessment. Provide numerous problem-solving opportunities throughout the semester—strive to include one problem-solving activity at each class meeting

SUMMARY

In summary, for learning to be complete, occupational therapy students must develop and utilize both explicit and tacit knowledge. Explicit knowledge is conscious knowledge used to name, describe, and organize concepts. Tacit knowledge is knowledge about patterns and relationships among elements in one's environment. It is acquired through day-to-day experiences without conscious effort. Instructors can meet the learning needs of students by designing, supporting, and arranging learning activities that promote the development and integrated application of explicit and tacit knowledge. With these types of learning experiences, students will be prepared to enter a profession and a health care environment that demand practitioners know "how" and "when" as well as "what" and "why."

REFERENCES

Baltes, P. B., & Baltes, M. M. (Eds.). (1990). Psychological perspectives on successful aging: The model of selective optimization with compensation. *Successful Aging: Perspectives from the Behavioral Sciences* (Ch. 1). New York: Press Syndicate of the University of Cambridge.

Lewicki, P. (1986). *Nonconscious social information processing.* Orlando, FL: Academic Press.

Reber, A. S. (1993). *Implicit learning and tacit knowledge: An essay on the cognitive unconscious.* New York: Oxford University Press.

Sheckley, B. G., & Keeton, M. T. (1997, May). *A review of research on learning: Implications for the instruction of adult learners.* Paper presented at the planning meeting of the American Association for Higher Education, Denver, CO.

Sternberg, R. J., Wagner, R. K., Williams, W. M., & Horvath, J. A. (1995). Testing common sense. *American Psychologist, 50*(11), 912-927.

POSITIVE REINFORCEMENT
Christina Griffin, MAEd, OTR

Educators need to be able to provide their own internal positive reinforcement for the quality and worth of their efforts and be able to wait for delayed reinforcement from others. In the clinic, the therapist gets positive reinforcement for a job well done on nearly a daily basis. This can be either from direct patient expression of appreciation or from seeing the daily progress patients make in therapy. An educator, however, has a different relationship with the students than the relationship between a clinician and a patient. The educator must take the lead in the teaching/learning process and be able to find satisfaction in doing this job well. Students do not generally give you positive feedback daily. In fact, you often get just the opposite; students will appear bored, not work as hard as they should, or actually challenge you on your course methods or grading. Many a professor has received a poor rating on anonymous student evaluations of courses for something the students requested in the first place. It is typical to receive compliments for the difference you made in the student's life long after graduation when actual employment as an occupational therapist suddenly makes your teaching relevant to your former student. If you are able to find self-satisfaction in the teaching role, then a career as an educator can be very rewarding and the delayed gratitude of graduates, now fellow occupational therapists, can be well worth the wait.

TEST QUESTION CLARITY
Christina Griffin, MAEd, OTR

Writing reliable and valid multiple-choice or true-or-false test questions can be very difficult. Enough information must be given to allow the student to formulate an answer, but not so much information as to give the answer away. The question stems and the answer choices must be clear and unambiguous. There must be one and only one correct answer. When writing questions, it is easy to make assumptions about the questions that students might not make. Students may interpret wording in a different manner than the writer intended and will frequently think of implications regarding the question that the writer had not intended.

I have found the following method very helpful in avoiding these problems and determining the students' real knowledge versus their test-taking "savvy." Although I usually score tests by machine from an answer sheet, I encourage students to write on the test papers to explain why they answered as they did for any question they were unsure of or felt was unclearly worded. They are to alert me to look for this explanation by writing "see # 2," etc. by their name on the answer sheet. If, after looking at their justifications for their answers, it is obvious that they understand the information but have missed the question due to a misinterpretation of what was being asked, I award the student the points. If it is clear that many students do not understand the question, then I can review it in class to ensure understanding of important material. This method helps me to discover misleading questions so that I can improve the question and increase the accuracy of my student evaluations.

PROFESSORS ARE FROM EARTH, TOO
Karen Sladyk, PhD, OTR, FAOTA

Every now and then, insert a family photo or vacation picture into your PowerPoint or slide presentation. This "alerting" activity calls students' attention back to the screen and helps them to understand their professor is a person of multiple occupations besides educator and researcher.

Reprinted from Sladyk, K. (2001). *Clinician to Educator: What Experts Know in Occupational Therapy.* Thorofare, NJ: SLACK Incorporated.

Chapter Three

ADULT LEARNERS AS COLLEGE STUDENTS

Marijke Kehrhahn, PhD

Over the past two decades, an ever-increasing number of adult learners have enrolled in college. The rising number of adults in the population, the economics of the current world of work, the explosion of technology, and the cultural value for life-long learning have resulted in an environment that presses adults into continuing their educations well beyond traditional school age. In 1999, the Council for Adult and Experiential Learning (CAEL) reported that "Adult learners are the new majority on many college campuses. Only about one-quarter of American college students attend full-time as residential students, while nearly half can be defined as adult learners" (p. 3). Unfortunately, many policies and practices in higher education have not been examined and refined to reflect today's college population (CAEL, 1999). Who are these adult learners in college? How are they different from traditional-age college students? How can faculty develop strategies that better meet the needs of adult learners in the college environment?

Adult learners are students who are 25 years of age and older and are financially independent of their parents (CAEL, 1999). Adult learners not only attend college classes and work toward degrees but also balance the demands of family, work, and community responsibilities. Adult learners have developed identities beyond the early-life role of student (CAEL, 1999) and have a wealth of experience from which they have gleaned many life lessons. Because of the unique nature of the adult learner in college, faculty teaching in higher education environments should actively learn about the needs of adult learners and develop strategies for supporting their successful participation.

ADULT LEARNERS BALANCE MULTIPLE LIFE DEMANDS

Adult learners balance the demands of higher education—class participation, reading, writing, homework, group projects, and communication with the instructor—with the ever-present demands of work and family. On any given day in the life of an adult learner, an ailing parent, a parent-teacher conference, a work emergency, or a school board meeting may take precedence over homework, studying, or even coming to class!

The most important strategy for supporting adult learners is having an understanding and respect for their personal life experiences and circumstances. The CAEL (1999) benchmarking study on adult–friendly higher education environments stated that flexibility was the most critical asset for adult learners. Be prepared to flex your course requirements, your timelines, and even your office hours to accommodate adult learners. Make sure that information about course requirements and assignments is available in multiple modes (written, electronic, and in class), that written information is explicit and complete, and that you are available to clarify expectations. Recognize that while traditional students may prefer face-to-face meetings during office hours, adult learners are likely to prefer telephone or e-mail conversations at a time that is convenient for them. You may want to consider developing "family-friendly policies" about class attendance and due dates, for example, excusing an absence for a child's spring concert or giving an extra day for completing an assignment when an adult learner has a big project due at work.

In addition to family and work demands, Cross (1981) found that institutional barriers—lack of access to campus offices and facilities, limited availability of information, limitations of student services for adult learners—often deterred adult learners from participating successfully in educational programs. You will find that adult learners will appreciate your ability to serve as a liaison to the larger institution. Try taking a part of a class session to generate a list of questions that students have about the school and then having students share answers. Develop an informal handbook of frequently asked questions (or have students do this for extra credit!) that you can share and add to each year.

ADULT LEARNERS ARE GOAL-ORIENTED

Adult learners tend to be more goal-oriented and goal-driven concerning their college educations than traditional-age students. Merriam and Caffarella (1999) reviewed a series of studies by the National Center for Educational Statistics that showed the vast majority of adult learners participate in education to advance in their jobs, secure a better job, or change careers. Working toward a degree or developing new professional skills almost always links to adults' future vision concerning their work, their family, and their financial future. In addition, adult learners finance their own education and may be receiving reimbursement for tuition from their employers. Some employers prorate the reimbursement rate based on grades. In summary, adult learners may see their education as much more of an investment and may see themselves as having much more at stake than traditional-age students. In order to teach adult learners effectively, faculty must understand and appreciate the goals and expectations of individual learners and establish a partnership with students that will lead to those goals being met.

Begin by finding out what the goals and expectations of your students are (Cross, 1981). While the best way to do this is to get to know each student individually, a large class may require a different approach. Develop a questionnaire that you can distribute to the students early in the semester. Ask questions such as the following: What do you hope to learn in this course? How will you use what you are learning now and in the future? What problems do you think you will be better able to solve once you complete this course? What do you expect from me as the instructor? What do you expect from yourself? From your fellow students? You may be surprised and even inspired by the goals of the learners in your class. Be frank with students about the degree to which you can deliver on their personal goals and expectations, but also be prepared to flex and individualize your course, your teaching, and your assignments to better match the goals of the learners.

ADULT LEARNERS BRING A WEALTH OF PERSONAL EXPERIENCE TO THE LEARNING ENVIRONMENT

Adult learners come to college with a wealth of personal experience which they have come to value as a source of learning. While traditional-age students may be content to soak in course content without question of its relevance or truth, adult learners are much more likely to question information that is presented and to look for its applicability in the real world. Research in adult learning has shown that experience is a critical pathway by which adults sort and value information and store it in memory for later retrieval (Merriam & Caffarella, 1999). Therefore, linking the learning in the classroom to experience is not only nice to do, but it is essential for effective learning to occur.

Use learners' experiences as a learning tool. Tennant and Pogson (1995) suggest that faculty must tackle two issues: How to get to know about learners' experiences and how to use experience to enhance instruction. To get to know more about the experiences of your students, develop activities that are designed to promote reflection on and articulation of what students have experienced and what they have learned. Test students' prior knowledge, formally or informally. Develop a pre-course questionnaire or ask students to submit detailed curriculum vitae (Tennant & Pogson, 1995). One experienced professor I know asks students to write letters to him about their past and current experiences and how they relate to the course content. These techniques not only help you understand the students' experiences but help students link new information being presented in the course to their current knowledge base.

Once you have become familiar with the experiences of the adult learners in your class, your task is not only to link the course content to their prior experience but also to challenge and expand students' understanding of their prior experience. One of the most effective ways of doing this is to encourage critical reflection on prior experience using new knowledge as an evaluative framework. Have learners select a problem from practice, or give them a detailed case study if their clinical experience is limited. Ask students to evaluate the problem by giving them specific questions on which to reflect. Having students complete this task in groups enhances their reflection and expands their knowledge by exposing them to multiple viewpoints and at the same time recognizes and values the various experiences of the learners. Once students have thoroughly explored the problem from their current knowledge base, provide new course content related to the problem. After students have had a chance to read about, listen to, and discuss course content, have them return to the original problem and reflect critically on it: What didn't they see the first time through? What did they learn in class that helps them see the problem differently? How did their clinical reasoning about the problem change with the addition of the new knowledge? How would they re-frame the problem to represent a more comprehensive understanding and a more effective solution? Finally, wrap up by asking students to generate examples of experiences from the past or experiences they expect to encounter in future clinical settings in which they will need the new knowledge they have gained in today's class. Creating this link from theory to practice is important to adult learners and critical for effective clinical instruction.

ADULT LEARNERS MAY HAVE BEEN AWAY FROM SCHOOL FOR SOME TIME

Many adult learners in college are finding themselves in formal learning environments for the first time in many years. This often means that adult learners may be wrestling with ghosts from their past schooling such as math anxiety or fear of failure, or they may bring inaccurate perceptions of what is expected based on high school or early college experiences. Adult learners who have been away from school for some time may be unsure of the standards, demands, and time requirements for successful course completion. Many adults come back to college with little experience or understanding of the current high-tech environment, and many return with rusty basic skills such as the ability to sit and read for 2 to 3 hours at a time, to write a research paper, or to take notes effectively. As the instructor, you can help by making expectations for the class explicit. What are your standards for written work? Provide models of papers that meet your standards. How much time should it take students to read this week's assignment? Give students a range of times, acknowledging that some students may need more time to read and process information than others. Generate class discussions that encourage students to share their struggles with completing assignments and strategies they have used to successful ends, highlighting the gap between what students may have thought they would have to do and what they actually had to do. This type of discussion helps adult learners develop more accurate perceptions of what is expected of them. In addition to what you can do within your own course, develop a working knowledge of the resources available at your college or university to help adult learners brush up their basic skills. Your college may offer a study skills workshop or on-line resources for writing standards. The student support center may offer one-on-one assistance with writing or math. Make students aware of these resources in general and discreetly recommend to individual students that they seek out additional support.

In addition, it is reasonable to assume that many adult learners who have returned to college are successful adults in other areas of their lives. They may find the college environment scary and confronting because it puts them in a position to have to prove their competence. They may expect more of themselves than they should because they have demonstrated competence in other areas of their lives. If their performance in class does not reflect the same high performance that they demonstrate in other areas of their lives, adult learners may become discouraged, upset, and may even look to blame the instructor for their lack of success. Cross (1981) suggests that building adult learners' self-confidence in educational experiences is important to their continued success. You can do this by encouraging adult learners to acknowledge conflicts between their identity as a competent adult and their difficulties with school work. Help them develop realistic expectations of their performance, and share your frustrations with your own performance when heading into new territory. Provide specific feedback on assignments and in-class performance, focusing on what the learner has done well and making concrete suggestions for improving future performance. Offer encouragement and support that will help the adult learner span the gap between adult life and academia.

ADULT LEARNERS ARE SAVVY CONSUMERS

Adult learners often work in service-oriented environments. Through their life experiences as consumers, they have come to expect a level of service that often exceeds the general standards in higher education. Adult learners know how much they paid for a course and they expect their money's worth! Adult learners will tend to see themselves more as peers of the instructor than of traditional-age students in the class and are likely to be more vocal than traditional-age students about their likes and dislikes concerning the course. Because of this different dynamic, teachers of adult learners must establish "adult" teacher-learner relationships (Tennant & Pogson, 1995) that are characterized by mutual respect, openness, and participation. Work to negotiate power and interests with adult learners in your class. For example, work with the class to determine how class time will be used and where emphasis should be placed in terms of content. Be clear with learners about content and competencies that are a required part of the curriculum and where flexibility exists. Encourage learners to take responsibility for establishing guidelines for class discussions and engage learners in solving class-related problems such as how to structure the class sessions so that each member has an opportunity to share his or her project. As the instructor, develop a healthy psychological climate within the classroom in which learners experience mutual respect, mutual support, and the freedom to say what they think and feel without being threatened. Demonstrate ways to value the input and experiences of learners in the class such as attentive listening to learner ideas and positive feedback for engagement in class discussions. Of course, conflicts may arise around issues that remain under the control of the instructor such as grading; these conflicts are best resolved in an atmosphere of mutual respect and understanding.

SUMMARY

As the number of adult learners who enroll in college continues to grow, college faculty will find themselves more and more engaged in establishing environments and practices in which adult learners will be successful. Fortunately, the fields of adult learning and adult education have much to offer by way of documented successful approaches to educating adult learners. By using some of the ideas presented in this chapter, you will become a more effective teacher of adult learners and will be well on your way to making the successful transition from clinician to educator.

REFERENCES

Council for Adult and Experiential Learning. (1999). *Serving adult learners in higher education: Findings from CAEL's benchmarking study* (Executive Summary). Chicago: Author.

Cross, K. P. (1981). *Adults as learners.* San Francisco: Jossey-Bass.

Merriam, S. B., & Caffarella, R. S. (1999). *Learning in adulthood: A comprehensive guide* (2nd ed.). San Francisco: Jossey-Bass.

Tennant, M., & Pogson, P. (1995). *Learning and change in the adult years: A developmental perspective.* San Francisco: Jossey-Bass.

STUDENT-DEVELOPED TEST QUESTIONS
Karen Sladyk, PhD, OTR, FAOTA

There are a variety of student-driven test question development ideas in the literature and in antidotal stories. Some suggest having students develop test or quiz questions as a way of making sure the students have done the reading assignments. Others suggest that student-developed test questions make the teacher's workload more manageable while helping students study the most important issues. One successful way of having students develop test questions can be used as a study guide for the whole class.

Instruct the students on what makes good test questions and how to write test questions with clarity and objectivity. Have each student develop one multiple-choice question for each lecture topic and one question for each related reading assignment, for example, one on the lecture of schizophrenia and one on the readings for schizophrenia. Have the students write a set for each topic covered on the test using the following format: Within the top inch of the paper, write your name and the answers to each question. Leave a one-inch space and then write each of the questions, marking it a lecture question or reading question. If many pages of reading are assigned, students can put a "page hint" next to their reading question.

Have the students pass the questions in daily as they go through the topics. Fold the top inch of paper down, covering both the student's name and the answers to the questions. Photocopy the folded page, resulting in only the questions showing. Bundle all the questions and put the resulting study guide on reserve reading in the library. The faculty can guarantee that a certain percentage of the test will be based on the study questions (generally 50% to 75%) or can give points for the development of test questions.

COLLECTING AND PASSING BACK PAPERS
Henriette Pranger, PhD

To avoid using too much class time calling out names to return assignments and collecting new assignments, I use a folding accordion pendaflex envelope (with the A to Z type labels) to collect and return papers and quizzes. The 26 tabs of A to Z are relabeled with each student's name, and students put their own incoming assignments in the correct section before class. After grading, the assignment is returned to the same section and the student picks it up before class. Empty sections clearly identify who did not turn in a paper.

Chapter Four

ACCOMMODATING COLLEGE STUDENTS WITH DISABILITIES

AN INSTRUCTOR'S RIGHTS AND OBLIGATIONS

Lori G. Sladyk, MS, CSE

As an occupational therapist, you are familiar with making adaptations to daily living tasks so that a client can be as independent as possible. You have undoubtedly discovered that there is often more than one way to complete an activity and still obtain favorable results. As an educator, you will be called upon to meet the needs of students in your classroom who have varying disabilities. How does one maintain the integrity of a program while ensuring that students leave class with the necessary tools and skills required to succeed as an entry-level occupational therapist? The purpose of this chapter is to highlight the laws that protect students with disabilities, to outline the responsibilities of educators in meeting student needs, and to discuss frequently requested accommodations.

BASIC LAW

Section 504 of the Rehabilitation Act of 1973 (Public Law 93-112) and the Americans with Disabilities Act (ADA) were designed to protect the rights of people with disabilities. Section 504 states that "No otherwise qualified handicapped individual in the United States shall, solely by reason of his or her handicap, be excluded from participation in, be denied benefits of, or be subjected to discrimination under any program or activity receiving federal financial assistance" (29 U.S.C. 794). The regulation applies to students who are "otherwise qualified" to participate in programs offered by postsecondary institutions that receive funding from the government. The handicapping condition must be one in which one of life's major activities, such as learning, is substantially limited. Handicapping conditions might include, but are not limited to, learning disabilities, speech impairments, attention deficit disorder (ADD), visual impairments, mental retardation, and psychological disabilities. The act mandates that institutions must provide appropriate accommodations and modifications to individuals so that equal access can be obtained.

Accommodations and modifications are expected to be reasonable and based on the needs of each individual with a disability. In other words, what might be considered an appropriate accommodation for one student may not be considered so for another student. Academic adjustments should provide the institution with a measure of the student's knowledge and skills that is equivalent or similar to assessments of other students (Brinckerhoff, Shaw, & McGuire, 1993).

Under Section 504, if a person believes he or she has been discriminated against on the basis of a disability in a program that receives federal financial assistance, the person may file a complaint with the Office for Civil Rights.

Each campus will have a 504 coordinator who generally does not work within the disabilities services office. The 504 officer is available to both students seeking accommodations and staff concerned with making accommodations.

STUDENT'S PERSPECTIVE

Many college students with disabilities have previously received services under the Individuals with Disabilities Education Act (IDEA,1990, Public Law 104-476) which applies to those between the ages of 3 and 21 (or upon high school graduation). This act guarantees that all students will receive a free and appropriate education in the least restrictive environment, and the burden is upon the school system to identify and provide services to such individuals. Under 504 and ADA, the individual is responsible for making his or her needs known through self-disclosure, for providing appropriate documentation of a disability, and for advocating for his or her rights. Many college-bound students with disabilities mistakenly expect a disabilities service provider on campus to serve in a capacity like their high school resource room teacher, providing content tutoring, assisting with homework, monitoring progress, and talking to instructors on their behalf

(Brinckerhoff, 1994). This can be a difficult transition for a student who has been in a protective environment.

During the first class, many instructors announce that students with disabilities are invited to make an appointment to discuss their needs as soon as possible. Some instructors place guidelines for students in their syllabus. An announcement is not required but may serve as a convenience for both teacher and student.

IMPLICATIONS

Under Section 504, individuals with a disability must initiate services or accommodations. Approximately 6% of all undergraduates report some form of disability (Henderson, 1995). Some colleges and universities have specific programs to address the needs of these students. Programs may include tutoring, counseling, study skills centers, summer institutes, seminars, and advocacy. Most programs have criteria for membership. However, to be considered for support services, the student must seek out the service and provide appropriate documentation of his or her disability. Students are responsible for speaking directly with instructors regarding their disabilities and needed accommodations.

ACCOMMODATIONS

Some students will know what accommodations they need based on awareness of their weaknesses and past experiences in the classroom. Other students will be less sure of their needs and may ask for accommodations that may not match their needs. For instance, a student with ADD who has difficulty tuning out extraneous stimuli might ask for extra time on an exam when in reality, the student might need to take the test in a separate, quiet room. The most common accommodations requested are as follows:

- Extended time: In most circumstances, 1.5 times the usual allotted time is considered reasonable. Some instructors elect to have the student start early so that class members finish at approximately the same time.
- Taped textbooks: The student is responsible for ordering his or her texts on tape, a service provided by Services for the Blind and Dyslexic. Because it may take lead time to prepare a book on tape, a student may ask which text you intend to use for an upcoming semester.
- Testing modifications: In addition to extended time, a student may need a test read to him or her, a scribe, or an alternate format on the exam. Additionally, a student may request to use a word processor, calculator, or spell-checker. Accommodations and modifications must be provided on an individualized basis. For instance, the use of a dictionary would not be appro-

priate for a test that measures vocabulary. A student who has a word retrieval difficulty would not necessarily need a calculator but may need access to a word processor with a thesaurus.

- Lecture notes: A student might ask the instructor for a copy of his or her notes or for an outline. Generally, students can photocopy a classmate's notes easily.
- Taped lectures: Many students with or without disabilities routinely tape lectures. If this makes you uncomfortable, you may dictate that students are allowed to tape lecture only and not ancillary discussions.
- Extended time on projects, papers, and presentations: In most instances, students are given several weeks to complete outside assignments, so extra time is not necessary if the student planned appropriately. However, if a student has several projects from various classes due on the same week, he or she may request an extension or opt to turn in an assignment early.

CONSIDERATIONS IN GRANTING ACCOMMODATIONS AND MODIFICATIONS

The law states that accommodations are to be reasonable and to ensure that students with disabilities have an opportunity to learn with their nondisabled peers. Because adjustments are determined on an individual basis, determining appropriate accommodations may seem overwhelming. Many postsecondary institutions have established policies for granting accommodations, modifications, course substitutions, program acceptance, priority registration, etc.

Begin by familiarizing yourself with your institution's current policies. Keep in mind that you have a voice in determining appropriate accommodations. In making adjustments, departments should determine the essential requirements of a program, the program's purpose, and the skills and competencies needed in the field following graduation (Scott, 1994). One student who was about to begin her level II fieldwork requested that her placement be within eight miles of her home because she had a learning disability. Her request was denied. If you are unsure or uncomfortable with a request, speak with the disabilities service provider on campus.

SUMMARY

As a postsecondary educator, you will undoubtedly teach students with disabilities. Some disabilities will be obvious, and some will go unnoticed unless disclosed by the student. The law dictates that otherwise qualified students will have an equal opportunity to learn as their nondisabled peers. Institutions are obligated to provide the accommodations that are requested to assist students. It is the student's responsibility to arrange for his or her needs. Accommodations are expected to be reasonable and not significantly alter the expectations of the program. Accommodations are made on a case-by-case basis. If you strongly oppose a modification, you may wish to discuss the case with your immediate supervisor or an on-campus disabilities specialist.

REFERENCES

Brinckerhoff, L. (1994). Developing effective self-advocacy skills in college-bound students with learning disabilities. *Intervention in School and Clinic, 29,* 229-237.

Brinckerhoff, L., Shaw, S., & McGuire, J. (1993). *Promoting postsecondary education for students with learning disabilities: A handbook for practitioners.* Austin, TX: Pro-Ed.

Henderson, C. (1995). Postsecondary students with disabilities: Where are they enrolled? *Ace Research Brief Series, 6*(6).

Scott, S. (1994). Determining reasonable academic adjustments for college students with learning disabilities. *Journal of Learning Disabilities, 27,* 403-412.

CLASS PORTFOLIO ASSIGNMENT
Christina Griffin, MAEd, OTR

As an educator, it is sometimes frustrating to receive calls from students on level II fieldwork asking for materials and references on topics that were covered in class (including handouts). Good intentions to be organized notwithstanding, most students complete only the assigned tasks due to time constraints. To spur ready access to clinical information, a portfolio of physical disability-related material, including class notes and handouts, is a required course assignment. Required categories are given to students who can then organize them in the manner they feel will be most beneficial to them. Most students use either a large notebook or a portable file case. Students receive a portion of their course grade for this portfolio. Grading is primarily on completeness, so not all material needs to be read by the instructor; thus, the grading is not very time consuming. Feedback from students on fieldwork has been extremely positive because reference materials are readily accessible and can be expanded easily with material learned at the fieldwork site.

EVALUATING RESEARCH PAPERS AND PRESENTATIONS
Karen Sladyk, PhD, OTR, FAOTA

Each faculty usually develops their own form for grading a term paper but at times wishes their form had more depth. Consider the following grading aspects for term papers collected from several peers:

- Clear definition of issue covered
- Literature supports the body text
- Personal information is labeled as such
- Length is appropriate to the depth of the topic
- Paper appears professional in presentation
- Student provides appropriate analysis
- Summaries present most important issues
- References are primary and not secondary or from the Internet unless appropriate

- Reliable research supports the problem
- Logical sequence
- Both sides of an issue are explored
- References are correctly cited
- Student followed outlined directions
- Grammar and spelling are correct
- Bridges help the reader move from topic to topic

Many of the same issues for papers can also be used for evaluating speaking or poster presentations. In addition, consider the following:

- Presentation is welcoming and inviting
- Professional appearance
- Does not read presentation
- Maintains eye contact with all of audience
- Introduces and summarizes well
- Uses research to support ideas
- Invites audience dialogue if appropriate
- Is not shaken by change of conversation

- States presentation objective
- Projects voice or idea
- Utilizes props or visual aids
- Professional posture and movement
- Stays within time limit
- Uses color or other visual effects as appropriate
- Clarifies misinformation
- Provides appropriate analysis

Chapter Five

GROUP DYNAMICS
IN THE CLASSROOM

Marijke Kehrhahn, PhD

INTRODUCTION

Group work is an important addition to your teaching repertoire because it promotes the kind of engagement, reflection, and dialogue that solidifies and embeds learning in a greater context and at the same time gives emerging professionals the opportunity to learn about working effectively in teams. Group work can be used within a single class period to promote content discussion, to get students engaged in solving a case problem, or to encourage the sharing of experiences and ideas. It can also be used over several class periods to organize students into teams that will work together to accomplish group projects, conduct group research, or make group presentations. Unfortunately, group work does not always result in high quality outcomes that are desired by teacher or student. What makes groups work? How can a teacher structure group work to maximize the likelihood that it will be an enjoyable and successful learning experience for students?

WHAT MAKES GROUPS WORK?

For groups to work effectively, they need to develop into a working team, manage the group dynamics, and clarify group tasks and individual member roles throughout their time working together. This formula for success sounds deceptively simple. Many professors do not attend to group processes at all when requiring group work in their classes. To maximize the value of group work, teachers should provide structure, activities, and support.

All groups need to develop into working teams to be successful. Tuckman (1965) established a framework for understanding team development that is still used extensively. His theory of group development includes four stages: forming, storming, norming, and performing. Groups go through the forming phase as members are introduced to each other and they become acquainted with the group task and timelines. Almost all groups then enter a storming phase when members struggle with each other to figure out how the group task will be accomplished and how they will work together. The norming phase happens when group members emerge from the conflict of the storming phase and come to agreement on how they will get their task completed, who will do what, and how they will work; they set norms (common expectations) for their group work. Once groups have set norms for their work, they enter the performing phase when they are able to work effectively. If you reflect on your own experience with group work, both positive and negative, you may recognize these developmental phases and may have insights into why certain groups did not work. Perhaps the group could not end the storming phase and agree on how the task would be accomplished? Perhaps the group set out to work without establishing mutual expectations which led to confusion and lack of coordination (Figure 5-1)?

In addition to group development, groups also experience interpersonal dynamics that can enhance or stymie the work of the group. For group work to be effective, group members need to get along well, communicate openly, and make individual contributions to the work. Common problems with group dynamics include members who cannot agree, members who are vying for leadership, groups that break into opposing subgroups and then gossip about other group members, and group members who are not pulling their weight to accomplish the group task. A group dynamics problem can have a small effect on a single class discussion group but can have a major impact on the success of a group project. On rare occasions, you may have to jump in and facilitate a group's resolution of the problem or dismantle a project group that cannot work well together.

The third important aspect of effective group work is task and role clarity. Often I have heard group members whispering among themselves, "What are we supposed to be doing?" Groups work more effectively when they are

Reprinted from Sladyk, K. (2001). *Clinician to Educator: What Experts Know in Occupational Therapy.* Thorofare, NJ: SLACK Incorporated.

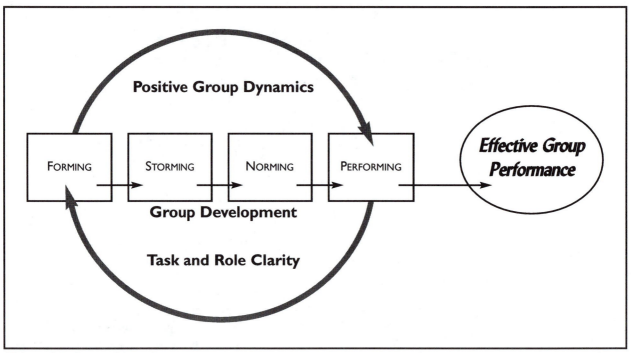

Figure 5-1. Successful work groups.

clear about how they should use their time and what outcomes they must produce. Knowing the roles that must be filled by individual group members (e.g., leader, recorder, timekeeper) also helps a group get off on the right foot. Groups that work together on a project over time need continuous structure and support; very few groups are effective at "running with" an unstructured task. As a professor, you should establish tasks, products, and roles in your lesson plans and provide written materials that clearly define tasks and group roles. These strategies save time and lead to on-target outcomes.

SUGGESTIONS FOR TEACHING PRACTICE

As the teacher, your planning and attention to group development, group dynamics, and group task can make or break the group work you have integrated into your curriculum. Here are some suggestions for designing successful group work.

- As you develop your curriculum, be clear about the purpose and outcomes of group work. Make sure you build in plenty of time for groups to work together during class sessions and develop materials that will support and guide group work.
- If you rely on group work as an important component of your teaching, teach a class session on how groups work. You can use the information provided here, have students discuss their best and worst group work experiences, and engage them in generating guidelines for effective group work. For most students, this knowledge of group process will be widely applicable in their professional lives.

- Provide a structure that will move groups through the developmental phases. For group projects, develop a worksheet and exercise that students can use in their first group meeting that promotes forming, storming, and norming. Provide a specific structure for group members to introduce themselves to the group (e.g., What strengths can you offer the group? What was your best experience in a group? Why? What was your worst experience in a group, and how would you fix what went wrong?). Provide key points about working together that the group must storm about and come to agreement on (e.g., Will we work together outside of class time face-to-face or via e-mail? Who will fill each role that has been described by the teacher? How will we handle disagreements?).

- For shorter group work, such as an in-class case analysis group, provide norms or expectations for how the groups will work together or have the entire class generate norms for how groups will work together at the beginning of the semester.

- Give groups an opportunity to assess their performance. An entire class can evaluate "How are we doing with group work?" based on the norms they set early in the semester. Follow up the evaluative discussion with an opportunity to generate improvement strategies. Do this about one-third of the way into the semester and group work will improve after this assessment.

Reprinted from Sladyk, K. (2001). *Clinician to Educator: What Experts Know in Occupational Therapy.* Thorofare, NJ: SLACK Incorporated.

- Develop a written assessment of group work so students who are hesitant to share negative reactions to group work feel more free to do so. You can summarize the comments from the written assessment and present them to the class for discussion.

- Provide project groups with a format for assessing their group performance. The format may be an informal discussion on specific points (e.g., How is our group doing at using our group time well? How are we doing with making decisions?), or it may be a written checklist that each group member fills out and turns in. A written checklist may ask group members to agree or disagree with statements about the group (e.g., Everyone is pulling his or her own weight to accomplish the group task) or to rate the frequency with which the group uses specific tools (e.g., How often does the group form an agenda prior to meeting? To what extent does one person lead the group discussion?). If a group is not working well together, you may need to step in and facilitate the discussion for them and make your own observations as well.

- Model good group process and demonstrate the use of strategies that help groups work effectively such as keeping to a time frame, explaining objectives for the group's time together, and debriefing a group discussion from the perspective of group process.

- Build group participation and performance into your grading scheme. Some professors ask group members to evaluate each other's participation and performance, develop scores associated with the feedback, and convert scores to points toward the students' final grades.

- Finally, provide groups with as much information and structure as you can. This includes written agendas for group meetings, worksheets to guide group discussions, evaluation forms for group work, samples of group products, and goals and objectives for the group. Creating written instructions and worksheets for groups may seem like overkill, but the documentation provides groups with something concrete to fall back on when they lose their way or disagree about tasks or expectations. Written instructions are especially important for groups that will be working outside of class time.

SUMMARY

Group work can provide exceptional opportunities for students to reflect on and engage with course content in a way that deepens their understanding and enhances their abilities to apply course content to a variety of situations. In addition, group work provides experiences from which students learn to work within a team, a critical competency for today's work environments. With thoughtful planning and teaching that incorporates knowledge of group process, the group work that you build into your curriculum can result in positive, multi-faceted learning for your students.

REFERENCES

Tuckman, B. W. (1965). Developmental sequence in small groups. *Psychological Bulletin, 63*(6), 384-399.

RECOMMENDED RESOURCES

Scholtes, P. R. (1988). *The team handbook*. Madison, WI: Joiner.

Silberman, M. (1990). *Active training: A handbook of techniques, designs, case examples, and tips*. New York: Lexington Books.

STUDENT ANGRY ABOUT A TEST QUESTION
Karen Sladyk, PhD, OTR, FAOTA

When an angry student approaches a faculty about grading on a test question, the student has generally had some time to think about the approach, but the faculty is often caught by surprise. If the problem is simple to correct, such as a math error, I handle it immediately. If more complex, I simply say, "OK, let me think about it, see me in my office at..." I have found that decisions I have made in an open classroom at the beginning or end of class are not always my best, and I deserve to give myself some thinking time.

"I DON'T KNOW WHY I GOT THE F—I STUDIED REALLY HARD!"
Karen Sladyk, PhD, OTR, FAOTA

Over time, I have come to understand that many people have different definitions of "studied really hard." I tell students that for every hour in class, 1.5 hours of studying/reading is expected as "homework." They usually agree that this is reasonable, however, are shocked when they calculate how many hours they should be studying if there are three equally spaced tests in the semester. A traditional three-credit class means 37.5 hours of class (50 minutes x 3 days per week x 15 weeks). That means about 20 hours of studying/reading per test.

Reprinted from Sladyk, K. (2001). *Clinician to Educator: What Experts Know in Occupational Therapy.* Thorofare, NJ: SLACK Incorporated.

Chapter Six

COLLABORATIVE LEARNING GROUPS IN THE CLASSROOM

Sherry Borcherding, MA, OTR

The peer group is a powerful influence that is not always utilized in teaching, yet we rarely work alone in a professional setting. One task every educator has is assisting students to move from viewing networking as cheating to viewing it as consultation or collaboration. Using a collaborative learning group in the classroom is one way to facilitate this shift.

Considerable research demonstrates that "collaborative learning produces higher achievement, more positive relationships among students, and healthier psychological adjustment than do competitive or individualistic experiences" (Johnson, Johnson, & Smith, 1991, p. iii). Bruffee (1987) asserts that learning is a social rather than individual event. In general, students learn critical thinking skills best in groups, talking to each other about biases and interpretations of material and events. Students working in small groups generate better quality ideas than students working alone, as students are stimulated by one another's ideas. Thus, the best way to increase the students' clinical reasoning, social maturity, and ability to make sound decisions may be through the use of collaborative learning groups.

Use of collaborative learning groups moves faculty from a position of "sage of the stage" to a position of "guide on the side"—a much more feasible paradigm in an age where no one can teach future professionals everything they need to know to practice. While the idea that faculty do not know everything can be disconcerting to some students at first, it is very empowering in the bigger picture. Students must be reacculturated from a traditional view of classroom authority resting with the instructor to a view that will grant authority to a peer instead. They must also be willing to exercise that same authority over a peer responsibly and in a friendly and helpful manner. Sometimes it takes a while for the students to reacculturate in this manner because the academic prohibitions against it are long-standing and thoroughly internalized (Bruffee, 1987). A student will typically say, "How do I know my classmate is right?"

The size of collaborative learning groups may vary from pairs to as many as eight students. Larger groups generate more ideas but less meaningful interaction. Groups larger than eight are no longer considered small groups. The optimum size for a group varies according to the situation and the task to be accomplished. The group becomes a team where each member develops a slightly specialized role, and more than one person may provide different kinds of leadership at different times.

There are several varieties of collaborative learning groups that can be used, from simple small group discussion in one class to a curriculum centered around problem-based learning. In the most basic group, students may discuss a topic proposed by the teacher and be asked to come to consensus, they may edit each other's writing, or they may develop and carry through assigned projects as a group. Because groups fall apart if they are not given a focused task, it is critical that the instructor provides a focus in the form of a task, question, or some clear topic of discussion.

The most basic collaborative learning scheme is that of breaking students into several small groups of three to five students to discuss a topic such as a reading assignment. In the small groups, students share ideas in answer to questions provided by the instructor. Before starting the discussion, it is best to tell the students how long they have to discuss and allow them to ask any clarifying questions they might have. The instructor circulates among the groups during the discussion. Roles may be assigned to each group member (e.g., facilitator, timekeeper, recorder, etc.). At the end of a given period (usually about 20 to 30 minutes), each group reports its consensus back to the collective, and the consensus from each group is discussed by the whole class during the last 15 to 20 minutes of the class.

In a collaborative group of this kind, students might be asked to discuss a reading assignment. Questions such as the following might be used:

- What was the author trying to say in the article?
- What concepts in this article did you have trouble understanding?
- Give an example from your own life where you have encountered a situation of this kind.
- How is this article useful in understanding the concept of human occupation?
- How does the Occupational Therapy Code of Ethics apply to this situation?

As each group reports back to the class, the instructor should refrain from commenting except to clarify. Responses may be placed on the blackboard or on an overhead. Students can be involved in discussing the differences between the ideas of various groups. Instructor insights can be added during the "teachable moments" that are created, but an instructor-dominated discussion should be avoided. Instead, redirect questions or comments to other students or ask open-ended questions that have no right or wrong answers (Myers, 1994).

Small discussions of this kind can also be used as a method of breaking up lecture time into smaller blocks of material so that it is more easily absorbed and retained by the students. After 15 minutes of lecture, 5 minutes of discussion can be inserted to revive the class and re-engage students in the material. Randomly assigning students into different groups each time groups are used broadens the range of perspectives the students encounter. One side benefit of this method of class discussion is that every student participates rather than only the more extroverted students.

There are many formats for collaborative learning groups. A slightly more complex strategy is that of a jigsaw puzzle. In this model, each small group discusses one part of the assignment, and then the students are regrouped so that each new group has one student from each of the original groups. Each person thus has something unique to contribute as the new group compiles the information needed. For example,

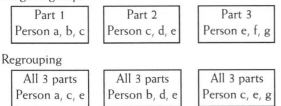

Original groups

Part 1 Person a, b, c	Part 2 Person c, d, e	Part 3 Person e, f, g

Regrouping

All 3 parts Person a, c, e	All 3 parts Person b, d, e	All 3 parts Person c, e, g

Two other examples of collaborative groups are structured controversy and roundtable. In a structured controversy, students assume different positions on controversial issues. A roundtable is a brainstorming technique in which students write in turn on a single pad of paper, sharing their ideas as they write. A variation of the roundtable is the round robin. Each person speaks in turn and no one speaks a second time until all have spoken. Having stu-

dents actively engaged with the class material rather than passively sitting through a lecture is an effective way to increase what is taken away from class each day.

When groups are working on long projects together (half a semester or longer), it is helpful to teach social and organizational skills by providing some measure of group process during the semester. Intervention may be necessary if the group process breaks down. When intervening in the process, however, instructors must be very careful not to intervene too early or too often so that groups do not become dependent on the instructor to intercede when inevitable conflicts arise. To facilitate group cohesion and interpersonal sensitivity, a group process assessment technique such as those suggested by Angelo and Cross (1993) may be used. In this way, the group is able to assume the responsibility of team building and autonomy by dealing with conflicts and other interpersonal problems. The group's members may be asked to complete the assessment individually and then to discuss similar and dissimilar responses of its members, followed by a report on how the group plans to deal with its problem areas (Walker, 1995). Conflict can be an important creative force, stimulating useful ideas and discussion, and should not be avoided by suppressing minority opinions (Myers, 1994).

Different students have different ways of contributing to the group. Whether or not the group assessment is utilized, a part of each student's grade is based on how well he or she works with others in the group. Another way of evaluating group interactions and each student's ability to carry a fair share of the work load is that of nominating. Each student nominates one person who was outstanding in the group and one or two others who were good. In this way, no student has to say anything negative about another student, but the final tally will show clearly which students participated and which did not (Matsuda, personal communication, May 1, 2000).

The largest obstacles to a good collaborative learning group are the instructor's need to be in control, a poorly designed task, and the belief that all relevant information is held by the instructor. Using collaborative groups frequently helps students become more comfortable with the process and with the idea that they can find information in other ways than being told by the instructor. Sometimes a group will have a difficult time getting started and will need to be stimulated by a few extra questions or by some additional piece of information. Most important is a positive atmosphere in which the students feel relaxed and unafraid of criticism (Myers, 1994).

SUMMARY

There are many benefits to using collaborative learning groups. Developing group skills is an accomplishment in itself. In collaborative groups, students also learn problem-solving and communication skills. Finally, active student involvement in maximizing their own and others' learning provides greater retention of the material and potentially greater student satisfaction with the class.

REFERENCES

Angelo, T. A., & Cross, K. P. (1993). *Classroom assessment techniques*. San Francisco: Jossey-Bass.

Bruffee, K. (1987). The art of collaborative learning. *Change, March/April.* 42:47

Johnson, D. W., Johnson, R. T., & Smith, K. A. (1991). *Cooperative learning.* Washington, DC: George Washington University.

Myers, R. L. (1994). *Cooperative learning groups: Making them happen.* Unpublished manuscript.

Walker, C. J. (1995). Assessing group process: Using classroom assessment to build autonomous learning teams. *Assessment Update,* 7(6):4-5

Chapter Seven

SERVICE-LEARNING
LINKING THE CLASSROOM TO PRACTICE

Anne Birge James, MS, OTR/L

Occupational therapy practitioners, educators, and students have been on a quest for the perfect occupational therapy program since the profession began. Practitioners often feel that students and new graduates are ill-prepared for the pace and complexity of entry-level practice. The pressures of current clinical practice require level II students and new graduates to possess effective professional behaviors and to understand occupational therapy theory in a clinically relevant way. Students believe that the academic portion of the curriculum contains insufficient "hands-on" experience to prepare them for level II fieldwork and entry-level practice. Educators agree that students need more clinical experience during their academic work in order to transition classroom skills more smoothly into the clinic. Practitioners, however, have little time for level I fieldwork students, and expanding clinical experience for pre-level II fieldwork students is often unrealistic.

One teaching option that addresses these issues is service-learning. Service-learning is defined as an active pedagogy where students are engaged in activities that both enhance the students' knowledge, skills, or perspectives and provide service to a community (Jacoby, 1996). Community is broadly defined and may include individuals in local neighborhoods; private or public organizations at local, state, and federal levels; and the global community through international organization or outreach programs (Jacoby, 1996). Although students may not be engaged in the specific practice of occupational therapy, they gain access to "real life experiences" that can enhance their level of comfort outside the classroom and facilitate the development of some crucial clinical skills. This paper will describe service-learning programs and highlight ways in which they can be used to 1) provide students with opportunities to interact with individuals of varied ages, ethnicity, socioeconomic status, health, and abilities; 2) promote students' understanding of and skills in client-centered practice; 3) promote reflective practice; and 4) facilitate students' professional behaviors.

ENHANCING PERCEPTIONS OF DIVERSITY AND DISABILITY

The "Standards for an Accredited Educational Program for the Occupational Therapist" (American Occupational Therapy Association, 1999) address issues of diversity, health and disability, and individual perceptions of quality of life. Students cannot appreciate the complexity of these topics through classroom experiences alone, particularly in programs where the student body lacks diversity. The broad definition of community in service-learning allows faculty to connect students with many populations, providing experiences that help them construct a richer understanding of people whose background and needs differ from their own. Examples of settings include senior centers, daycare centers, programs for single mothers, supported employment, day treatment centers, homeless shelters, schools, group homes, welfare-to-work programs, hospitals and clinics, advocacy groups, and diagnostic-specific agencies (e.g., the Multiple Sclerosis Society).

Service-learning opportunities with people with disabilities provide students with an opportunity to enrich their "textbook image" of varied disabilities to develop a better understanding of the range of abilities that may be found in individuals with specific pathology. For example, students enrolled in a course focused on work-related programming were involved in a service-learning assignment with a local school district whose students were placed in supervised work settings. Direct involvement with teens with cerebral palsy provided the occupational therapy students with an image that reinforced and expanded upon the descriptions of cerebral palsy they had read about. Experience seems especially important in helping students see that a diagnosis does not present uniformly across individuals. Students then learn to use the diagnosis as a guide for anticipating a range of possible deficits, preventing them from making assumptions based on a stereotypic image that may lead to ineffective or incomplete evaluation and treatment choices.

DEVELOPING COLLABORATIVE SKILLS FOR CLIENT-CENTERED PRACTICE

Reciprocity between the server (student) and the person or group being served is at the core of service-learning (Jacoby, 1996). The service provided is determined collaboratively, but the needs of the community are determined by the members, not the server (Jacoby, 1996).

Reciprocity also eschews the traditional concept of volunteerism, which is based on the idea that a more competent person comes to the aid of a less competent person...Service-learning encourages students to do things with others rather than for them. (Jacoby, 1996, p. 8)

Many students enter their occupational therapy program with the notion that they will "help" or "do to" the client, which is consistent with a traditional medical model of care. The more holistic approach to care embraced by occupational therapy, however, requires students to learn to actively engage clients in the intervention process. Experience in service-learning helps students learn important collaborative skills. Students must learn to engage community members in a dialogue to determine their needs, articulate the skills they have that may help meet those needs, and work collaboratively to develop an appropriate plan of action. These are basic skills used in a client-centered approach to occupational therapy and are steps that are fundamental to the occupational therapy assessment and planning process.

The opportunities for student learning in a truly reciprocal service-learning experience are great; however, careful planning is required to match student learning needs with the needs of the community being served. The following example illustrates what can happen when a reciprocal relationship is not established. A group of students in the work-related programs course mentioned earlier were placed in a sheltered workshop program for adults with varied disabilities. The workers were paid for simple assembly work based on the amount of work they completed. A letter had gone to the agency prior to confirming placement that described the types of skills that students might use that could both serve the agency and meet the students' learning goals. Learning goals were broadly defined in order to be flexible but included the application of occupational therapy skills to facilitate the work-related programs within the agency. The agency indicated an interest in having students; however, when the students began, it became clear that their defined needs fell outside of the learning goals of the course. Students helped the agency by serving lunch and snacks to the client-workers but were discouraged from any interaction with clients at work or alteration of work stations. Supervisors were concerned that the students might interfere with productivity, which was directly linked with the workers' payment.

Students were frustrated as they observed workers in poorly designed work stations who could benefit from ergonomic assessment and modification, yet those directing the program defined the agency's needs, so students were limited to tasks that did not provide them with an optimal learning experience. Discussion between the faculty and the agency regarding service needs, rather than a brief correspondence via mail, could have determined whether reciprocity was possible or the placement was simply inappropriate for the course objectives.

DEVELOPING REFLECTIVE PRACTITIONERS

Experience is the basis for gaining knowledge through service-learning, however, experience alone is insufficient. Reflection on experience, framed by learning goals, is necessary for learning to occur (Jacoby, 1996; Morton, 1996). Reflection is a mental activity used to give meaning to experience. Kolb (1984) described the process of reflection as being crucial for embedding a concrete experience in memory through abstraction. Without abstraction, the experience is not transformed into knowledge that can be applied to problems in the future. It is not only experience then, but how that experience is reflected on that contributes to learning. Students engaged in service-learning should participate in a variety of reflective activities with opportunity for feedback including journal writing, course discussion, and written or oral assignments. For example, students engaged in service-learning for the course focused on work-related programming used journals, class discussion, and a poster presentation to describe how occupational therapy principles were used (or could be used) to meet the needs of the community in which they served. Reflection combined with faculty and peer feedback often helped students see possibilities that they had missed, which enhanced their understanding of occupational therapy in work-related settings.

Occupational therapy practitioners also use reflection. A reflective stance toward practice is essential for the development of clinical reasoning skills necessary for effective occupational therapy practice. Reflective service-learning assignments can help students develop valuable reflective skills that enhance both life-long learning and clinical problem solving. Faculty feedback facilitates students' development of deep and effective reflective skills and helps students see connections between their service and the course objectives (Morton, 1996).

DEVELOPING PROFESSIONAL BEHAVIORS

Professional behaviors are attributes that, while not explicitly part of a profession's theoretical or technical base, are necessary for success in the profession (May, Morgan, Lemke, Karst, & Stone, 1995). These attributes include commitment to learning, interpersonal and communication skills, effective use of time and resources, use of feedback, problem solving, professionalism, responsibility, critical thinking, and stress management (May et al., 1995). Service-learning provides students with an opportunity to develop these skills (Jacoby, 1996), which are difficult to learn in a classroom setting. For example, students engaged in service-learning in work-related programs initiated contact with the agency to which they were assigned, collaborated with the agency to complete a needs assessment, articulated the occupational therapy services that might be used to meet those needs, provided a service, and assessed the results. In addition, students managed the logistical demands such as scheduling and transportation. Several of the experiences included additional challenges such as conflicting service and learning needs (described earlier) or agencies whose identified needs seemed ambiguous and unclear to the students.

Increased attention has been given to the development of professional behaviors in occupational therapy curricula. Traditional academic assignments provide faculty with little opportunity to critique skills in this area, making it difficult to give students concrete and constructive feedback. Students often see their classroom behavior as separate from their clinical behavior and do not view feedback regarding classroom behavior as relevant to their clinical performance. Service-learning provides students with an opportunity to practice professional behaviors and receive feedback in environments that better approximate practice settings. Use of structured feedback sheets can help individuals in the community provide students and faculty with feedback specific to professional behaviors. Students can be encouraged (or required) to establish goals related to professional behaviors to be addressed in subsequent service-learning settings. Multiple service-learning experiences throughout the occupational therapy curriculum can provide students with opportunities to respond to feedback and improve professional behaviors, addressing deficit areas before they enter level II fieldwork.

PRACTICAL ADVICE

There are many resources available to help faculty establish effective service-learning programs. The best place to start is within one's institution. There has been an increased interest in and commitment to community service by universities across the country and an increase in the incorporation of service-learning into curricula. Many colleges and universities have departments that are responsible for establishing and promoting community outreach, including service-learning. These departments have established relationships with community agencies and can often provide assistance with determining community needs, scheduling students, and program evaluation.

The effectiveness of any service-learning assignment will be enhanced with some careful planning up front. Mintz and Hesser (1996) describe five Critical Elements of Thoughtful Community Service initially developed by the Campus Outreach Opportunity League:

1. Community voice: The needs of the community to be served are determined by the community rather than the students serving. Clarification of community needs by faculty facilitates a good match between community needs and course objectives.

2. Orientation and training: Students should receive an orientation to the community they are to serve, including the culture of the community and their service needs.

3. Meaningful action: The service must be necessary and valuable to the community so that students feel they have made a difference and their time was well spent.

4. Reflection: This is a crucial component to learning. Reflection should occur soon after the experience and help students to place their experiences in a broader context.

5. Evaluation: This should measure both the impact of the experience on student learning and the effectiveness of the service in the community. Evaluation is crucial for developing and maintaining an optimal experience for both the student and the community served.

SUMMARY

Service-learning has wonderful potential for enhancing occupational therapy education. Students enjoy well-designed service-learning experiences and feel they contribute significantly to their learning. Additionally, the university provides a needed service to the community in which it resides, making service-learning a win-win opportunity for all involved.

REFERENCES

American Occupational Therapy Association. (1999). Standards for an accredited educational program for the occupational therapist. *American Journal of Occupational Therapy, 53*, 575-589.

Jacoby, B. (1996). Service-learning in today's higher education. In B. Jacoby & Associates (Eds.), *Service-Learning in Higher Education: Concepts and Practices* (pp. 3-25). San Francisco: Jossey-Bass.

Kolb, D. A. (1984). *Experiential learning.* Englewood Cliffs, NJ: Prentice Hall.

May, W. W., Morgan, B. J., Lemke, J. C., Karst, G. M., & Stone, H. L. (1995). Model for ability-based assessment in physical therapy education. *Journal of Physical Therapy Education, 9*, 3-6.

Mintz, S. D., & Hesser, G. W. (1996). Principles of good practice in service-learning. In B. Jacoby & Associates (Eds.), *Service-Learning in Higher Education: Concepts and Practices* (pp. 26-52). San Francisco: Jossey-Bass.

Morton, K. (1996). Issues related to integrating service-learning into the curriculum. In B. Jacoby & Associates (Eds.), *Service-Learning in Higher Education: Concepts and Practices* (pp. 276-296). San Francisco: Jossey-Bass.

E-MAIL JOURNALING
Nancy Dooley, MA, OTR

In the occupational therapy assistant program at New England Institute of Technology, we have had great success in using electronic communication for reflective journal writing for fieldwork students. During the past year, we have required students to use e-mail to keep interactive and reflective journals of their thoughts and experiences on fieldwork. We have used this method in level II fieldwork to help keep in touch with students we are supervising in community practice sites such as adult daycare centers and a shelter for homeless families.

The students have had a positive response to e-mail journals because it provides an efficient way to give and receive feedback in a very timely manner. The clinical educator can respond at his or her leisure to questions and concerns that arise in the clinical setting, especially on days when the educator is not present. When students work in collaborative pairs, they may share journal entries with each other as well as the clinical educator. The clinical educator, in turn, may choose to reply to both students at once or to each individually. E-mail seems to provide a forum for expressing opinions and personal reactions to clinical situations that is less threatening than face-to-face conversation.

We have also required e-mail journaling for our students during level I fieldwork in community-based and traditional settings. The journals are part of a 1-hour-per-week seminar that accompanies the actual fieldwork experience. For educators trying to read and comment on the journals of several students each week, it is much less cumbersome than passing notebooks back and forth. The journals also force students to think about their fieldwork experiences before coming to the seminar. The educator has also responded to the journal entry, usually asking additional questions or suggesting learning activities. This quick interaction tends to produce a higher level of discussion during the seminar's limited meeting time.

Reprinted from Sladyk, K. (2001). *Clinician to Educator: What Experts Know in Occupational Therapy.* Thorofare, NJ: SLACK Incorporated.

Chapter Eight

THE BULLETPROOF SYLLABUS

Karen Sladyk, PhD, OTR, FAOTA

- *What I said in class:* "Use any style you want for this paper."
- *What I meant:* I do not care if students used APA, MLA, or any other footnote or reference style.

- *What they heard me say in class:* "Use any style you want for this paper."
- *What they thought I meant:* Do whatever style you want, including no style or one you invent yourself.

The title of this chapter is a bit misleading because at best your syllabus will be bullet-resistive, but the concept of bulletproofing is a worthy goal. I use the analogy of bulletproofing because every teacher has a class where someone will attempt to intercept (shoot at) your syllabus, usually the assignments, to benefit his or her grade.

Because many universities and colleges view the syllabus as a contract between the teacher and student, considerable time should be spent in preparing this "contract." Brinckerhoff, Shaw, and McGuire (1993) identify the minimum requirements for a user-friendly syllabus as follows:

- Title, course number, professor's name
- Required texts
- Purpose of course
- Objectives
- Course requirements
- Grading policy
- Format for each topic, date, reading, purpose, study questions

When you develop your syllabus, consider the following suggestions:

1. *Always follow the college policy on syllabi.* A teacher cannot expect support from administration on a syllabus issue if the syllabus does not follow school rules. If the college policy has weaknesses, ask to be on the revision committee.

2. *Take time to be reflective on your own androgogy.* Pedagogy is how we teach children; androgogy is how we teach adults. Understand how your teaching style will affect your syllabus development before you begin to write it.

Colleges usually have policies that require a syllabus be given out in the first week of class. Because all teachers will want their syllabus copied at the same time, there will likely be a backup in the copy center. To have reflective time and your syllabus ready for copying, you will need to start developing it at least 4 weeks before it is passed out.

3. *Ask peers for samples of their syllabi.* This is especially helpful when you are taking over an existing class. Samples give you syllabus ideas you want and do not want. Ask OT peers and non-OT peers to review your final draft for clarity.

4. *Include the basics.* Course title, course number, room, professor's name, and contact information are the basics. Additional information such as section number, time, office hours, required textbooks, and department name will be helpful. It is not atypical for a student to come into your first class, sit there, and then discover they are in the wrong class after you passed out the syllabus.

5. *Include a list of outcome objectives.* "By the end of the semester, the student will be able to..." Some faculty begin with the objectives and design the course tasks around the objectives. Other faculty design the tasks first and then write the objectives. Some OT departments have written class objectives as a committee and expect the educator to meet these objectives.

Just like in the clinic, objectives need to be measurable and outcome-oriented. Check with the program director to see what program evaluation plans might be tied to your specific courses.

Reprinted from Sladyk, K. (2001). *Clinician to Educator: What Experts Know in Occupational Therapy.* Thorofare, NJ: SLACK Incorporated.

When designing objectives, consider the level of the course. For example, introduction class objectives may use words such as identify or demonstrate. Higher level classes may use analyze or integrate. Use *Taxonomy of Educational Objectives* for a guide (Bloom, 1956).

6. *Include a list of class policies.* It is the policy section that makes your syllabus bullet-resistive, but this is not effective if you do not follow your own policies. Word spreads very quickly in a class if one student is given an exception.

   A. *Consider allowing students to develop the class policies.* On the first day of class, present your list of policies/objectives and invite the students to participate in developing a class culture. Encourage both sides of an issue such as losing points for lateness or computer printer problems. Update the list and give students back the finalized policies the following class.

   B. *Begin the policy section with a list of the generic department policies.* For example, if the department has a policy that students call the secretary if they will miss class, then include this. Include the college's policy on special accommodations regarding the Americans with Disabilities Act.

   C. *Consider attendance policies seriously before initiating them.* Although it is educationally sound that a student is present for all classes, attendance policies can be difficult to manage. If the class objectives are demonstrated by a student, then his or her attendance is not an issue unless peer projects are effected. Attendance tracking requires faculty time; on the other hand, no one wants to be treated by an OT or OTA who did not go to class.

   Whether attendance is mandatory or not, include a statement emphasizing that if a class is missed, the student is responsible for getting all notes and handouts from a peer. This will put the responsibility on the student and avoid students in your office asking you to repeat everything they missed in class.

   D. *Make late assignment policies very clear.* Our department requires that all late assignments be attached to a department form that requests permission for the assignment to be accepted late. The faculty decides if the reason for lateness is acceptable and what points, if any, are lost. These forms are stored in the student's department record and patterns for consistent lateness are documented.

   An assignment is late if it is turned in past the first 10 minutes of the class it is due. This policy was put in place when as a faculty, we saw students cutting class to finish their work and racing to class in the last 10 minutes to turn in the assignment. This was inherently unfair to those who had completed the assignment and attended class.

   E. *Have a policy for missed exams.* We use the same form for missed exams as for late assignments. One professor I know allows any student to miss any exam without permission even if they feel they are "not ready." Students know ahead of time that all makeup exams are scheduled for the afternoon of the last day of final exam week. Needless to say, a student very rarely misses an exam.

   F. *State a policy on individual and group work.* Make clear the differences between "assistance and collaboration" and "unethical" work.

   G. *State a policy on typing.* Whenever possible, have all assignments typed because handwriting slows the correcting process down significantly. Sloppy handwriters will argue that the reader did not read the answers correctly. Additionally, typing eliminates many errors and improves professionalism.

   H. *Make a statement on syllabus changes.* Consider adding statements such as the following: "The syllabus is subject to verbal adjustment at the discretion of the faculty. Although the syllabus provides most information on assignments, many details are covered in class. Only consistent class attendance will provide you with the information you need."

   I. *Expect students to keep a photocopy of all assignments turned in.* From time to time, assignments get misplaced by the faculty or the student. A faculty can expect that a copy of a missing assignment could be turned in within 24 hours. If the student is not on campus the next day, I ask him or her to e-mail or traditional mail me the copy (postmarked within 24 hours).

   One way to avoid the problem of a student not passing in the assignment and then saying he or she did is to count the number of papers in class and then count the number of students present. I do this only when I'm having a problem with missing papers.

7. *Provide a section on assignments.* This syllabus section is what the student wants to read most because it includes the work and value of the work to be completed. To encourage higher level learning, the assignments should be varied, allowing each different learning style to be utilized and practiced. Provide as much detail as possible to reduce students' last-minute questions they want answered the night before an assignment is due.

   Consider your other class loads and other responsibilities when developing the due dates. If an assignment is large and comprehensive, consider student due

Reprinted from Sladyk, K. (2001). *Clinician to Educator: What Experts Know in Occupational Therapy.* Thorofare, NJ: SLACK Incorporated.

dates for assignments in classes taught by other faculty. For everyone's mental health, avoid due dates when other classes also have large projects due. If an assignment is large, consider collecting the assignment in smaller sections over time. I generally have big assignments due before holiday weekends so that students are free to enjoy the holiday, and I have flexible correcting time. This is especially true over the Thanksgiving weekend.

8. *End the syllabus with a schedule of topics and readings.* Providing an entire semester schedule helps both the student and faculty stay focused. Staying on schedule assists the students in meeting the outcome objectives. Including the reading assignments allows students to read before and after the topics are covered in class. The faculty should check and double check the dates on the schedule and allow for campus days, midterm break, and special fieldtrips. In addition, be aware of possible illness or snow days.

REFERENCES

Bloom, B. (Ed.). (1956). *Taxonomy of educational objectives.* New York: McKay.

Brinckerhoff, L. C., Shaw, S. F., & McGuire, J. M. (1993). *Promoting postsecondary education for students with learning disabilities.* Austin, TX: Pro-Ed.

SERIOUSLY SILLY STUDY AIDS
Karen Sladyk, PhD, OTR, FAOTA

Many antidotal stories are available about ways to have students study especially boring but important information such as medical terminology or muscle origins/insertions. Several educators use different versions of the same creative exercise that follows.

Have students in small groups develop a skit, game, poem, song, dance, or other presentation (perhaps a puppet show) that covers some of the material to be addressed on the final exam. A few days before the exam, have each group present their theatrical event to the class. Laughter and silliness raise the class spirit while increasing class bonding and offering different study approaches in the usually stressful period of final exams.

Another version of this exercise has the students building study aids with food, for example, mapping the sections of the brain on a head of cauliflower. It is amazing what students can do with gelatin or assorted raw vegetables. The added benefit is an automatic buffet for the end of class.

Grading can be for creativity and depth of topic covered. A small percentage of the test grade can be awarded.

NOTES ON READINGS
Karen Sladyk, PhD, OTR, FAOTA

One frustrating issue that affects many educators is knowing that some students do not read the supporting materials assigned to a particular lecture topic. This is sometimes made worse when the students tell the teacher that they did not even buy the book. Often, idealistic threats that there will be test questions based on the readings do not even motivate students. Consequently, the teacher is faced with how to develop a value in reading as well as making sure the student masters the reading content.

One way to encourage reading is to have open notebook quizzes that are based on the reading. Students can make any notes they want from their reading and use these notes during designated quizzes, but use of the textbook is not allowed. Quiz questions should be varied, including multiple choice, short answer, and short essay. Students not only read the chapters but also develop better note-taking strategies. In addition, these book notes make excellent reviews for the National Board for Certification in Occupational Therapy exam.

Reprinted from Sladyk, K. (2001). *Clinician to Educator: What Experts Know in Occupational Therapy.* Thorofare, NJ: SLACK Incorporated.

Chapter Nine

MULTIPLE USE OF STUDENT PORTFOLIOS

Henriette Pranger, PhD

Students can develop portfolios to enhance their college experience. This chapter describes three types of portfolios that you could encourage your students to develop: the learning portfolio, the employment portfolio, and the prior learning assessment (PLA) portfolio.

Learning portfolios focus on the student's course and fieldwork experiences. The portfolios are often required for course completion or program completion. The use of student portfolios enhances the student-teacher connection. Research suggests that the process of creating a portfolio enhances student learning of the subject matter (Sheckley & Legrow, 1999).

The format of student portfolios includes a physical binder or on-line website that highlights and summarizes the student's learning. For a course portfolio, the teacher provides students with written learning outcomes that help determine the portfolio's content. The teacher may also show students an example "learning essay" along with a list of possible types of supporting documentation. Ideally, the teacher would provide a link to the assignment description and sample portfolios as part of the course's website.

An exit or employment portfolio is another option for students. The institution's program guidelines serve as the organizing principle for the student's portfolio. Students often begin the portfolios as part of a reflection seminar in their junior or senior year and then continue to add information as coursework and fieldwork are completed. The

organization of an employment portfolio is important, and students may want to discuss the format with professionals in their field prior to presenting the portfolios as part of their employment interviews.

PLA portfolios are slightly different from the portfolios described above. The PLA portfolios are created by adult students returning to college. PLA portfolios document learning acquired from work or other life experiences prior to the adult's enrollment in college. The portfolios are evaluated for college credit. The credit award shortens the adult's time to degree, saves money, and prevents the adult from repeating courses in areas in which he or she has already acquired college-level learning. Published guides to this type of portfolio development (Lamdin, 1997) or assessment (Whitaker, 1989) are available from the Council on Adult and Experiential Learning.

REFERENCES

Lamdin, L. (1997). *Earn college credit for what you know* (3rd ed.). Chicago: Council for Adult and Experiential Learning.

Sheckley, B. G., & Legrow, M. (1999). The educational benefits of completing a portfolio of prior experiential learning. *Learning Experience Trust News* (London, England), pp. 2-3.

Whitaker, U. (1989). Assessing learning: Standards, principles and procedures. Chicago: Council for Adult and Experiential Learning.

Reprinted from Sladyk, K. (2001). *Clinician to Educator: What Experts Know in Occupational Therapy*. Thorofare, NJ: SLACK Incorporated.

Chapter Ten

USING LISTSERVS TO ENHANCE FIELDWORK EDUCATION

Brenda Smaga, MS, OTR/L

During level II fieldwork, it is advantageous for faculty to communicate with students and for students to network with each other. An electronic mailing list, more commonly referred to as a listserv, may be used as an alternative communication and educational tool during fieldwork. The listserv format proves valuable in encouraging frequent communications and networking between all students on fieldwork. There are both formal and informal communications that allow students to continue relationships established in class and provide support for each other. For the instructor or academic fieldwork coordinator, this easy method of quick and timely communication helps to address issues students are experiencing. Educationally, topics and cases may be discussed between members, allowing students to experiment with different treatment methods and approaches while on fieldwork.

WHAT IS A LISTSERV?

A listserv is a group of e-mail addresses that allows sending the same communication to all addresses in the group using one unique address, sometimes referred to as the command address. Listserv was developed by Eric Thomas in 1981 to handle distribution of messages through Bitnet, and Bitnet remains a major listserv management program (Gilster, 1995).

There are two broadly defined types of listservs: asynchronous and synchronous. In an asynchronous listserv, the listserv manager sends the e-mail to all the members, but the members cannot reply and thus cannot communicate back to the sender. In this type of listserv, the members do not know how many or who is on the listserv and they do not have communication abilities with each other. In some asynchronous listservs, it is possible for the person to reply to the listserv manager, but this is usually through another e-mail address and typically for changing an address or deleting a name. This type of listserv is excellent for sending fliers for information about events, articles for self-study, information on a topic of interest, or advertisements of travel bargains and new books. In *BeginnerNet in Rehabilitation* (Pomeroy, 1997), there is a comprehensive listing of newsgroups, a type of bulletin board/listserv of interest to occupational therapy.

Synchronous listservs provide a unique group e-mail address for any member of the group to use to communicate to the whole group. In this type of listserv, there are two ways to communicate to the group. One is to address e-mail using the group's address such as "OT Stars," and the other is to reply to e-mail sent by someone in the group. This type of e-mail is accessible through any e-mail account and does not require full Internet access. When a person replies to e-mail sent to the command address, everyone on the listserv gets the message. Some students are confused by this and think they are replying only to the individual who sent the e-mail. This can cause some embarrassment. In a synchronous listserv, members can identify who they are in their communications to each other, but their personal e-mail addresses are not available to listserv members. The listserv manager is the only one who will have this information and be able to communicate to individual members. This type of listserv lends itself to discussion about a particular topic and sharing of information where comment and networking is encouraged. Many clubs, community groups, and organizations use this type of listserv.

HOW DO I BEGIN?

A suggested sequence would be to:
- Investigate various listserv websites and your college's server capabilities to support a listserv.
- Create the listserv and make yourself manager or chief editor.
- Create a course outline with assignments and deadlines, seeking student input about frequency and type.

Reprinted from Sladyk, K. (2001). *Clinician to Educator: What Experts Know in Occupational Therapy.* Thorofare, NJ: SLACK Incorporated.

- Train the students prior to fieldwork in how to use the listserv, giving them actual experience. Define the rules!

- Update a comprehensive member list for both faculty and students.

- Monitor e-mail at least every other day to provide timely replies. Save, comment, and track e-mail communication.

- Evaluate successes and failures with an informal request for feedback and a more formal end-of-the-fieldwork evaluation.

WHAT ARE MY CHOICES OF WEBSITES?

There are general and educational websites that offer free listserv services. www.egroups.com is a general site that provides a range of services for both small and large listservs and is easy to navigate. It allows for a private listserv that is not open to public members. As with other commercial sites, it adds advertisements to your e-mails. www.blackboard.com is a commercial site that is used by educators. This site offers free on-line courses on various teaching methods using technology. Taking a course would help a beginner instructor to see how to incorporate different types of assignments into a course.

Colleges, other than your own, also offer listserv services. www.lsoft.com/lists/listref.html is a major listserv resource and can link you to the college listservs available (L-Soft International, Inc., 1996). They have directories of existing listservs. Your college may have listserv capability and can customize your listserv needs. Colleges using recent versions of Lotus Notes now have the capability to develop a linked hierarchy of listservs for single or multiple classes.

HOW DO I CREATE A LISTSERV?

Detailed information on how to create, control, and manage electronic mailing lists is available in a manual published on-line at www.lsoft.com. But to start, this is more than you need. After you have chosen the server site, you should follow its simple directions. The basics are to choose a name for your listserv. Try a catchy name such as "otstars." This will be the command name of your group, and the e-mail address will be otstars@egroups.com. This is the e-mail address the manager and group members use to send e-mail. You will then be asked to write a brief description of your group such as "OT students on level II fieldwork."

Somewhere in this beginning process you will need to select a password. Having multiple passwords may confuse those of us with the best of memories, so choosing one for all your occupational therapy accounts is usually a good idea. The next step is to indicate options, and this is where you want to choose the private group option over a public

group option. Also, choose the option making it mandatory for people to apply for membership, so you can catch a changing address. There are other choices, but skip those in the beginning. The final step is to create the list of addresses. The list does not care if a name is attached to an address or to whom the address belongs. If you want to add a name, follow the address with parentheses and insert the name there as in this example, bsw@msn.com (Bonnie). This helps during the back and forth communication on the listserv to quickly identify the sender. When you complete the list, be sure you have added your own address, both college and at home, if you want to access the list from both places. You will get duplicate messages, but it is more convenient.

The final touch is to indicate that you are manager of the list. A symbol will be added next to your address to indicate you are chief editor or manager. You are now ready to send a message! As manager, you may do this in two ways: one is directly from the website menu and the other is from your home or work e-mail server.

WHAT SHOULD I INCLUDE IN THE COURSE OUTLINE?

This modified course outline should include deadlines for assignments stated in terms of date and time such as Sunday at 10:00 p.m. The list of dates for an e-mail to be sent to the group should include not only assignments but other communications. A general description of the fieldwork facility, questions about the certification exam, and graduation requirements could be scheduled general communication topics. Reminders about graduation deadlines, a member's birthday, or other important dates or events can be sent on-line. Most listservs allow you to type out a list of reminder e-mail and schedule the dates in advance.

Short assignments are best for listserv format. Besides case studies, assignments may include presenting an ethical issue, a multicultural issue, describing the team meeting, the coordination of services, the COTA and OTR working relationship, or providing a sample of documentation styles with a sample note. Students like to share new types of treatment techniques they have learned or what it was really like to do a particular evaluation. *Assistive Technology for Persons with Disabilities* (Mann & Lane, 1995) has a fairly complete index of networks that have bulletin boards and databases, and some offer free electronic mail services.

WHAT PRIOR STUDENT TRAINING IS REQUIRED?

The semester prior to level II fieldwork is an opportune time to teach students how the listserv will be used and for students to practice using it. Prior training will enhance the quality of the students' output and will also jump-start students who are reluctant to engage in the process. Ask all students to bring their current e-mail address and show them how the listserv manager creates the main listing in a computer lab session. Then have students enter their own profiles, if it is available, by accessing the website that will be used in the future. This will give them experience in navigating the website and finding their listserv.

When the listserv is thus established, all the students can practice by sending messages to the group using the group's listserv address. Try a focused topic such as "What do I fear most about fieldwork?" during this practice session. Students should practice attaching and detaching documents from e-mail because you will probably send your comments to students this way.

WHAT ARE THE LISTSERV RULES?

Most listservs establish rules that govern what is permitted on the listserv. Banned most often is offensive language, shouting through the use of all caps, advertising your own work or others', and repetitive messages such as a thank you or "I agree" that clutters up your mailbox. In addition, students should not forward spam mail, chain letters, or Internet hoaxes. Refer to the comprehensive rules provided by the American Occupational Therapy Association's listserv for examples of other dos and don'ts.

HOW MUCH INFORMATION ABOUT STUDENTS SHOULD BE SHARED?

In the semester before fieldwork, it is a good idea to begin a list of all the students with names, home addresses, fieldwork addresses, telephone numbers, fax numbers, and e-mail addresses. With the students' permission, this list should be made available to faculty and fieldwork students. Include a list of faculty e-mail addresses other than the listserv manager. Students like to contact faculty when they have questions about clients and cases in their sites, and the faculty love hearing from them directly. After fieldwork is over, it may be desirable to add the career coordinator at the college to continue communications with the students about job postings. Students might find it helpful to get messages from the registrar and dean of students about graduation and transcripts for licensing. These people should not be members, but their messages may be forwarded to the group.

HOW OFTEN? HOW MUCH?

Some students will require more help than others during fieldwork. The instructor may need to set limits for some or encourage and provide frequent support for others. In this mode of teaching, it is easier to personalize the pace and amount for each student. Your comments and feedback will encourage reaching and accepting challenges at that student's level of ability. Short responses that include a question about what you would do next or how it could be different would help students explore other possibilities.

Because student assignments are "open to all to view," there is peer pressure to do one's best, too. A list should be used to track completion of assignments and grades just as for any class. In this format, having students complete a minimum of 80% of the assignments helps those who have difficulty accessing their e-mail. It will give students choices on assignments they like to do and an opportunity to ignore topics in which they are not interested. Forwarding e-mail to other faculty with particular areas of expertise enhances the quality of feedback to students. Saving printed copies of assignments in a notebook by student names makes it easy to refer to past messages. Saving your replies is essential if contention or confusion arises. At times, you will want to refer to these in planning future courses or doing research about on-line education.

WHAT ARE THE LIMITATIONS?

Students who are not comfortable with technology will not like this form either. Students who are not fast typists have found this a tedious method. Students should be encouraged to write no more than two paragraphs. Unless the assignments are required for class credit, some students will never be heard from unless they have a problem and need help. Conversely, some students who like attention frequently write asking for lots of responses from everyone. For the instructor, managing a listserv may be time-consuming. Some students will need to change their address with each placement and some will use public library computers. Encouraging students to use universal e-mail addresses such as juno.com or hotmail.com will limit the number of changes. Printing e-mail is time-consuming but a good idea for the first time or for selected communications such as specific assignments. Some sites will have a saving feature for your use.

HOW DO STUDENTS USE THE LISTSERV? WHAT DO THE STUDENTS LIKE?

Most students will follow the deadlines and assignments consistently. Some will ignore what they do not want to do and participate in what they want. Some students add fun items such as poems, greeting cards, and funny antidotes about their experiences in the clinic. Encouraging these communications adds to the fun and keeps things light and collegial. On the other hand, when serious fieldwork concerns and family tragedies surface, students will give support to one another that is both

Reprinted from Sladyk, K. (2001). *Clinician to Educator: What Experts Know in Occupational Therapy.* Thorofare, NJ: SLACK Incorporated.

encouraging and wise. Listserv communications help to alleviate the aloneness that many feel after being so close on campus. Students will also e-mail the instructor privately, rather than use the listserv, if they do not want everyone to know their issue. This is a helpful option, and the listserv should not be used as a substitute for confidential communication.

Foremost, students enjoy the communication frequency. They enjoy quick access to the instructor to answer questions and get advice. They enjoy quick access to each other to keep up on news and share experiences. Students comment frequently about the value of case studies and find it interesting to read each other's cases. For many, it gives them ideas for treating their clients, but mostly they are just fascinated by the variety of experiences.

REFERENCES

Gilster, P. (1995). *The new Internet navigator.* New York: John Wiley and Sons, Inc.

L-Soft International, Inc. (1996). *General user's guide to listserv, version 1.8c.* (On-line). Available: http://www.lsoft.com/manuals /index.html.

Mann, W. C., & Lane, J. P. (1995). *Assistive technology for persons with disabilities.* Bethesda, MD: American Occupational Therapy Association.

Pomeroy, B. (1997). *BeginnerNet in rehabilitation.* Thorofare, NJ: SLACK Incorporated.

LIVE VIDEO AS A LABORATORY PRESENTATION AID

Jeffrey L. Boss, MS, OTR, and Nancy A. Everhardt, MOT, MEd, OTR

Demonstrating small activities such as knitting or finger goniometry can be difficult when dealing with large groups of students. To resolve this, we use live video in ways similar to those seen on "how-to" television shows. An 8-mm video camera/recorder is mounted on a cart-based stand (Figure 10-1). The mount allows the camera to rotate and tilt, as well as allowing a height adjustment of about 18 inches. The stand also holds a 27-inch monitor, which keeps cables from being a safety hazard.

We position the camera behind and above the seated demonstrator (Figure 10-2) to provide the students with an over-the-shoulder view of the activity. This view is the one they will have as they perform the activity with others. The camera (Sony TRV-25) has a 64X-zoom feature that facilitates a very close-up view; however, at high zooms, it is difficult to stay within the camera's field of vision. We recommend outlining the camera's view area in tape on the tabletop to guide the demonstrator's movements. For a crisp image, ask the demonstrator to slow his or her movements to prevent blurring.

Using live video has the advantage of immediacy as compared to using videotaped demonstrations of an activity:

- Immediate responses to students' questions without having to stop and rewind the tape.

- Various views of the activity offer more in-depth explanations.

- When students demonstrate advanced knowledge, it is easy to omit or adjust parts of the demonstration.

The equipment is readily available or easily justifiable for a multiplicity of uses. Feedback from students indicates a preference for live video presentations over taped. Use of live video appears to reduce the number of repetitions required for the demonstrations, thereby saving time and instructor fatigue.

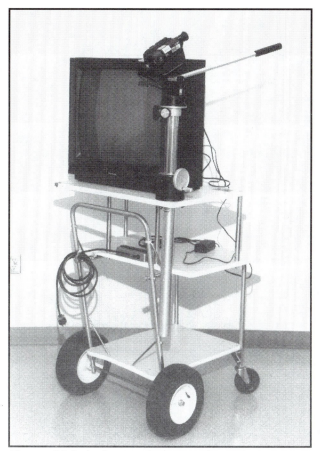

Figure 10-1. An 8-mm video camera/recorder is mounted on a cart-based stand.

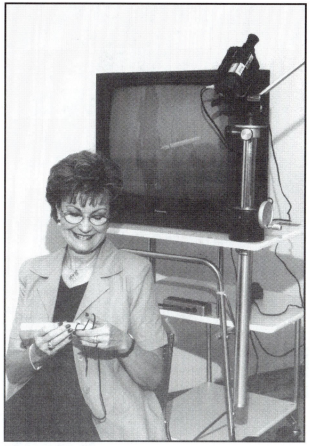

Figure 10-2. The camera is positioned behind and above the seated demonstrator.

TECHNICAL GLITCH CARDS
Sherry Borcherding, MA, OTR

What it is: A Technical Glitch Card (Figure 10-3) is like a "get out of jail free" card that allows a student to turn in one assignment late due to a computer malfunction with no questions asked and no excuses needed.

Why it is needed: Whether you are teaching by distance learning or just reading assignments typed on the computer, there are always excuses, sometimes very legitimate, for students not getting papers in on time due to problems with the computer. "The dog ate my homework" has now been replaced by "The server was down when I tried to dial into the chat room" or "I had it written on time, but the printer in the computer lab was off-line when I went to print it this morning." It is impossible to know whether the various reasons given are valid or not and a waste of time to try to figure it out. In an effort to be fair to students who have legitimate computer problems and avoid rewarding students who have creative minds for good excuses, one useful strategy is that of providing each student with a Technical Glitch Card.

How it is used: Under this plan, one assignment during the semester may be turned in late without question or penalty by attaching the card to the assignment. The date and assignment are noted on the card. Besides being easier for the instructor, the card gives the students who are less technically proficient a sense of security around computer malfunction. Rarely are the cards used, but when they are used, they are a straightforward method of handling late assignments.

Figure 10-3.
Sample Technical
Glitch Card.

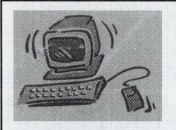

205 Loss & Disability
Technical Glitch Card

This card is good for one, unpenalized, late assignment due to computer problems.

Specify below which assignment was delayed due to unforeseen computer problems and turn in to Sherry for the assignment to receive full credit.

Name: _____

Assignment: _____

Due Date: _____

Reprinted from Sladyk, K. (2001). *Clinician to Educator: What Experts Know in Occupational Therapy.* Thorofare, NJ: SLACK Incorporated.

Chapter Eleven

AN ASSIGNMENT LINKING THEORY TO MISSION AND PHILOSOPHY DEVELOPMENT

Vicki Smith, MBA, OTR/L

Occupational therapy educational programs are required to meet the Accreditation Council for Occupational Therapy Education Standards (American Occupational Therapy Association [AOTA], 1999). These standards include ensuring that the student is able to plan, develop, and organize the delivery of services to include the determination of programmatic needs such as staffing and service delivery options and develop strategies for effective use for professional and nonprofessional personnel. The standards also require students to understand how history, theory, and sociopolitical climate influence practice (AOTA, 1999).

An assignment that is used to foster student skills in programmatic development is to have the student develop mission and philosophy statements for either a medical model-based program or a nontraditional program that provides (or has the potential to provide) occupational therapy services. This type of exercise can also foster the integration of theory principles as they relate to the occupational therapy service needs of the program being evaluated or developed. The assignment provides a working outline that instructors can use to help guide the students in developing mission and philosophy statements which includes a practical exercise for guiding theory integration into the philosophy development.

Development of a mission statement for occupational therapy services needs to be guided by the mission statement of the corporation or organization through which the services are being provided. The organization's mission statement provides the occupational therapy professional with guidelines of the business activity of the organization, including staffing, resource allocation, programming, and services provided (AOTA, 1996). These defined guidelines are then integrated into the occupational therapy mission statement and further developed into the philosophy of services provided. Philosophy development is guided by choosing occupational therapy theories that effectively provide services identifed by the mission statements (Figure 11-1).

This exercise begins with the instructor providing a brief scenario of a program situation that needs to have programmatic issues addressed. The scenerio should give basic information about the clients served, goals of the organization, and program environment. For example, this paper will outline the process of writing a mission and philosophy outline for the following scenario: Occupational therapy is managing an aquatics program that is part of a community-based, nonprofit organization.

The purpose of a mission statement is to guide and define an organization's business activities and to identify a shared view for the company's desired transformation process (AOTA, 1996). An effective mission statement is approximately one paragraph written in 10th grade language, has a vision for about 5 years of anticipated growth, and is a group effort from all employees working in the department or organization. This builds a shared commitment among the staff for providing high quality services, ensures that the employees understand why the program exists, and defines the therapist's role in the department (Umiker, 1998).

One method that can be used for developing a mission statement is to answer these questions:

- Who are we?
- What do we want to become?
- What are our guiding objectives (Hellriegel & Slocum, 1989)?

Figure 11-2 provides an example of an outline for a mission statement created for an aquatics program.

A philosophy statement is used to further define the therapist's beliefs about the program and its services. A program philosophy can be developed by answering the following questions:

- What is our professional philosophy?
- What are our beliefs about the program?
- What can we accomplish?
- What are the theoretical bases for the program?

Reprinted from Sladyk, K. (2001). *Clinician to Educator: What Experts Know in Occupational Therapy*. Thorofare, NJ: SLACK Incorporated.

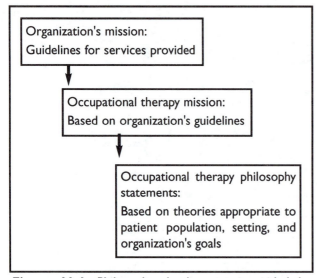

Organization's mission:
Guidelines for services provided

Occupational therapy mission:
Based on organization's guidelines

Occupational therapy philosophy statements:
Based on theories appropriate to patient population, setting, and organization's goals

Figure 11-1. Philosophy development is guided by choosing occupational therapy theories that effectively provide services identifed by the mission statements.

Who are we?
- Occupational therapists/professionals
- Part of an interdisciplinary team
- Specialists in aquatics therapy

What do we want to become?
- The leading providers of aquatics therapy to orthopedic/neurological clients
- Outpatient-based therapy treatment providers
- Treatment providers to ages ranging from young adults to geriatrics
- Providers of high-quality, efficient services

What are our guiding objectives?
- Community-based treatment
- Service the community support groups

Figure 11-2. An example of an outline for a mission statement created for an aquatics program.

Choose a few theories for the program design that represent the clients served and the services provided. Emphasize that students do not want to choose just one theory, or the program will be very limited in its scope of practice. Likewise, if too many theories are chosen, the department's treatment approach will be too broad. Figure 11-3 provides an example of an outline for a philosophy statement created for an aquatics program. Once the outline has been completed, the students are asked to develop these concepts into a statement form generally consisting of two to three paragraphs. The beginning of the philosophy should read as if the statement "We believe" is at the beginning of the document.

Students often ask for more guidance for theory choices. Some guidance tips include the following: Look at the population that was defined in the mission statement; if it is a neurological population being served, start with the theories that address neurological deficits and build from there. Another question often asked during philosophy development is, "If we do not choose a particular theory, does that mean it cannot be used as an evaluation and treatment method in our department?" A good response is that the set of theories defined in the philosophy is used as a guide to the department's beliefs about the services provided, not a complete list of all services provided. Any theory can be used as long as it is appropriate for the individual client and does not differ too much from the philosophical base of the program.

Completed mission and philosophy statements are not provided to the students. It is recommended they do research and find mission and philosophy statements on their own through contact with businesses, hospitals, and organizations or through the Internet and develop their own style for final-

izing their statements as they relate to their individual clients, reimbusement agencies, and consumers. Suggested grading guidelines can be viewed in Figure 11-4.

This assignment can be completed individually or in a group format. It also provides a basis of information that can easily lead to other management task assignments such as fiscal and capital budget development and development of outcomes programs.

SUMMARY

A hands-on approach to developing a program's mission statement and philosophy allows students the opportunity to apply management theory to real-life problems. It also provides guidance and a practical example of how to link occupational therapy treatment theories into program designs. Students report that the assignment is difficult, but it is an opportunity to apply their knowledge to a practical situation. This assignment helps them visualize how occupational therapy concepts are organized in order to provide high-quality services to a variety of customers.

REFERENCES

American Occupational Therapy Association. (1996). *The occupational therapy manager.* Bethesda, MD: Author.

American Occupational Therapy Association. (1999). *Standards for an accredited educational program for the occupational therapist.* Bethesda, MD: Author.

Hellriegel, D., & Slocum, J. W. (1989). *Management.* Reading, MA: Addison-Wesley Publishing Co.

Umiker, W. (1998). *Management skills for the new health care supervisor.* Gaithersburg, MD: Aspen Publication.

An aquatics therapy program can help clients:

- Alleviate pain
- Enhance functional independence
- Decrease neurological abnormalities (Bobath, PNF, NDT theories)
- Increase orthopedic functioning (biomechanical theory)
- Decrease stress (wellness theory)
- Create a sense of identity and responsibility (Model of Human Occupation)

Figure 11-3. Example of aquatics program philosopy outline.

Mission Statement

• Does the statement follow the organization's goals?	1	2	3
• Does the statement answer the following questions:	1	2	3
• Who are we?	1	2	3
• What do we want to become?	1	2	3
• What are our guiding objectives?	1	2	3

Philosophy Statement

• Theories chosen reflect the needs of the population served.	1	2	3
• Theories chosen reflect the goals of the organization.	1	2	3

Statements Review

• Statements are written in 10th grade language.	1	2	3
• Statements document a vision for growth.	1	2	3

1=information/question not addressed
2=information/question somewhat addressed
3=information/question clearly addressed

Figure 11-4. Grading guidelines.

MAKING PROGRAM DEVELOPMENT MEANINGFUL TO STUDENTS

Karen Sladyk, PhD, OTR, FAOTA

Management classes often have students develop new occupational therapy programs on paper to demonstrate the process of program development from philosophy through ordering supplies. After understanding needs assessments, students begin their design with a mission statement and philosophy of their new program. A bit dry and often without meaning, these topics can lose the students' attention quickly. After a few minutes of introductory lecture to introduce language, I put students into small groups of five to eight students. All the married students form one group, the single men form another, and the single women are asked to form in small groups of friends. I then ask each group to write a group philosophy for dating beginning with "Dating is..." and to follow that with a mission statement, "We believe..."

It is amazing what each group comes up with, usually funny, but clearly demonstrating the different ways a philosophy and mission statement can be written. The groups read each statement, and I list on an overhead key phrases that can be moved from the dating mission statement to a program statement. Possible frames of reference on dating are discussed. Problems are addressed when two frames conflict such as when two people dating conflict on their missions. The students leave with a personal understanding of philosophy, mission statements, and frames as well as a list of phrases that could be used in their program development project.

Reprinted from Sladyk, K. (2001). *Clinician to Educator: What Experts Know in Occupational Therapy.* Thorofare, NJ: SLACK Incorporated.

Section Two

MANAGING AN ACADEMIC CAREER

Chapter Twelve

THE TEACHING PORTFOLIO

Henriette Pranger, PhD

"Save everything," advised a senior faculty member during my first year teaching. Her advice was based on years of chairing the retention and promotion committee at her college. Some colleges now require faculty to develop teaching portfolios as part of the promotion or job application process. Every teacher saves the occasional student letter or other testimony of teaching effectiveness, yet those documents are not enough to create a teaching portfolio.

A teaching portfolio summarizes and highlights a teacher's career (Edgerton, Hutchings, and Quinlan, 1992; Urbach, 1992); therefore, a wide range of documentation is needed. In the past, portfolios were maintained in a three-ring binder separated by tab indexes. In addition to maintaining a binder, some teachers place their portfolios online; that is, they create an individual website with links to specific portfolio sections. This chapter describes what documents should be included in a portfolio.

CONTENT GUIDELINES

Individual institutions generate portfolio content guidelines; however, teaching portfolios generally document 1) teaching accomplishments, 2) research and scholarly activity, and 3) service. Specific portfolio documentation differs from discipline to discipline and from individual to individual. Portfolios of occupational therapy professors would include documentation of their clinical practice, fieldwork supervision, professional association activities, and related publications and research.

The first section of a teaching portfolio introduces the reader to the teacher. Most portfolios begin with a table of contents. An electronic portfolio might begin with a simple web page that could contain the teacher's picture and links to the portfolio sections. The first section also includes biographic material such as a curriculum vita (CV), statement of the portfolio's purpose, and a summary of the individual's teaching philosophy. Table 12-1 indi-

cates additional documentation that a teacher might include in the remaining sections.

Another section, included either at the very beginning or end of a portfolio, is a narrative called "Goals for the Future." If included in the beginning, consider also writing an introduction to each portfolio section that explains how the proceeding documentation relates to your philosophical beliefs and personal goals.

PORTFOLIO ORGANIZATION

As you review portfolio examples, you will quickly discover organizing strategies that separate effective from ineffective portfolios. For example, if you decide to create an on-line portfolio, resist the temptation to merely upload all the existing files and scanned documents. What is visually appealing and effective in a physical binder is overwhelming when presented on-line. If you are still in doubt after reviewing some on-line examples, read the literature on what makes an easy-to-read web page (e.g., www.smartcomputing.com).

The concepts of reliability and validity can be used to determine how much documentation to include. Reliability refers to obtaining similar results on repeated measures of learning. Anything documented is stronger when evidenced by two to three different sources. For example, including sample student work along with your grade book would be stronger than just including your grade book.

Validity refers to whether or not the measurement technique measures or validates the purpose; therefore, documentation from external sources strengthens any documentation that you create. For example, the inclusion of an organization's marketing tool in addition to listing an external presentation on a CV strengthens the validity.

The evaluation of the overall portfolio's content is conditional upon its purpose and the specific outcomes the

Reprinted from Sladyk, K. (2001). *Clinician to Educator: What Experts Know in Occupational Therapy*. Thorofare, NJ: SLACK Incorporated.

TABLE 12-1		
SUGGESTIONS FOR DOCUMENTATION		
Teaching Accomplishments (Skills and Outcomes)	*Research and Other Scholarly Activity*	*Service*
Course syllabi	Annotated bibliography	Awards, honors, grants
Current teaching schedule	Current research projects	Committee activities
Evaluation summaries (student/peer)	Publication copies	Membership/leadership in academic/ service organizations
Example of PowerPoint presentation	Seminar/conferences	
Fieldwork supervision	Agendas/certificates	Participation in radio/TV programs
Level I site feedback	Textbook development	Professional consulting
Level II completed FWEs	Presentation handouts	Clinical practice
Grade distributions	Supervision of theses and	Service on editorial board or
Information on course development	dissertations (e.g., signature	publication reviews
Link to student project websites	pages, abstract)	
Sample assignments		
Sample of student work with instructor comments		
Student letters/testimonials		
Teaching innovations		
Use of instructional technology		

portfolio is designed to document. Specific assessment criteria should be gathered from research conducted at your institution. For example, you may want to meet and discuss your department's evaluation criteria with your supervisor. You would then use those criteria as the organizing principles of your portfolio.

RESOURCES

Resources on portfolio development include published books (Seldin, 1997), examples of hardcover portfolios, or electronic portfolios. Examples of electronic portfolios are found by simply keying in "Teaching Portfolios" in your favorite search engine. Journal articles are also helpful (Cox, 1995; Zubizarretta, 1994.). Additional on-line help includes college resource centers with links to individual college assessment guidelines, example portfolios, and other helpful websites.

FINAL ADVICE

The advice to "save everything" should serve you well whether or not you are ready to create your own portfolio. Both scan and save documents on disk or preserve documents in plastic. Consider becoming proactive in your

efforts and always be on the lookout for creative ways to document your career. For example, ask for two copies of the agenda when you present at a conference, one to write on and one for your portfolio. Finally, be prepared to revise your portfolio each semester as part of your self-evaluation process. As long as you teach, your portfolio will be a work of art "in progress."

REFERENCES

Cox, M. (1995). A department-based approach to developing teaching portfolios: Perspectives for faculty and department chairs. *Journal on Excellence in College Teaching, 6*(1), 117-143.

Edgerton, R., Hutchings, P., & Quinlan, K. (1992). *The teaching portfolio: Capturing the scholarship of teaching.* Washington, DC: American Association for Higher Education.

Seldin, P. (1997). *The teaching portfolio: A practical guide to improved performance and promotion/tenure decisions* (2nd ed.). Boston: Anker Publishing Co.

Urbach, F. (1992). Developing a teaching portfolio. *College Teaching, 40*(2), 70-74.

Zubizarreta, J. (1994). Teaching portfolios and the beginning teacher. *Phi Beta Kappan, 76*(4), 323-326.

THE EDUCATOR'S FOUNDATION RÉSUMÉ
Karen Sladyk, PhD, OTR, FAOTA

A foundation résumé is a master résumé of everything professional in your career. As soon as you start or even begin to think about starting an academic career, begin a foundation résumé on computer. This foundation résumé will house all of your professional data and will be used to make shorter versions of other résumés or CV. Make a goal to update the foundation résumé every 3 months to avoid forgetting about items that could be included.

Formats of a foundation résumé are varied but should include the following:

- Education
- Academic experience
- Presentations
- Research projects
- Registrations/certifications
- Committee work

- Clinical experience
- Publications (journals, books, other)
- Professional associations
- Funded grants
- Dissertation/thesis committees
- Conferences

A new faculty member will likely not have some areas filled, but the foundation résumé is only a storage site to cut and paste to other résumés. The foundation résumé should store all information, so you should not delete data. For example, the presentation section may go on for 15 years and information may be outdated, but do not remove it. There may be a time when you will need to check old information, and the foundation résumé is a record of professional events. Also, a foundation résumé provides a place to reflect on lifetime professional development.

There will be many requests for updated résumés and CV (shortened academic-focused document) during an academic career. Often, conference committees will request a résumé or CV before a speaking engagement. Promotion or retention committees may also request a résumé or CV. State or national associations may need a CV to allow a person to serve on a committee or to qualify for awards such as FAOTA. The foundation résumé provides the blueprint and storage area to make these special-request résumés look complete.

TO PHD OR NOT TO PHD?
Karen Sladyk, PhD, OTR, FAOTA

Many occupational therapy and occupational therapy assistant departments have faculty trained at the master's level. Some universities will not consider a faculty candidate unless he or she has completed or is near completion of a doctorate degree. Many colleges will hire at a master's degree but expect faculty to continue school while teaching, a sometimes difficult task. Before accepting a new teaching position, have a good understanding of what continuing education is expected to maintain the job and what requirements are needed for tenure.

Many different doctorates are available, including the traditional research-based PhD and the project-based EdD. ScD and clinical or law doctorates are also available. With the growth of the Internet, distance doctorates are now available from accredited universities. Research all doctoral-level programs available to you to find one that lights your passion. There is no doubt that doctoral-level work will improve your thinking and your teaching, not to mention the profession as a whole.

The bottom line is that each faculty must first evaluate his or her career goals before deciding on pursuing a doctorate. Check with faculty from the college or university you might be interested in teaching at to find out if one degree is preferred over another or if one type is considered unrelated.

Reprinted from Sladyk, K. (2001). *Clinician to Educator: What Experts Know in Occupational Therapy*. Thorofare, NJ: SLACK Incorporated.

Chapter Thirteen

UNIQUE TIME MANAGEMENT OPPORTUNITIES FOR FACULTY

Karen Sladyk, PhD, OTR, FAOTA

This chapter is written, light in heart, in an attempt to put the time management issues facing new faculty in perspective. It is interesting how people outside of academia view academic time management, as illustrated by the following stories.

I am reminded of a candidate we invited to apply for a new faculty position who apologized for not having the time to send an updated résumé (she had sent an old one). I thought, "If she does not have time to send a current résumé, she has no clue how to manage the first few years of being an occupational therapy educator." She was not offered an interview.

Further, family and friends will think you have more time than ever because now you "get summers, just about all of January, and March break off." Even supportive parents view your job as "cushy." What others do not see and often cannot understand is the enormous amount of hours that go into preparation and correcting. Preparation is even more acute in the first few years of teaching. Just when you feel you have mastered your current responsibilities, the occupational therapy faculty will vote to gut the curriculum in favor of a new approach and you will start all over again.

Actual teaching is just one aspect of your position. Advising week typically arrives at the same time as major papers need to be graded. Then you may have open houses on weekends, homecoming, occupational therapy club activities in the evening, and committee work, not to mention that you need to publish and present papers in your area of expertise. Why would anyone want to become an occupational therapy educator? The personal and professional advantages outweigh the heavy workload.

Occupational therapists are usually very good at time management because of our skills in analyzing tasks and activities. We have the basic understanding of time management concepts as part of our clinical practice. But the academic career concepts are different from the clinical career, as I have attempted to illustrate in Table 13-1 of stress levels in a typical semester.

This is not to say that people do not have additional stressors, but the table attempts to illustrate that although a clinician's work is stressful, it typically stays steady over time while a faculty's stress periods have extreme ups and downs. This extreme movement up and down can be exhausting by itself because adaptation is difficult to achieve. This is why time management is essential to faculty.

Mackenzie (1997) suggests in his bestselling book, *The Time Trap*, that people should start with an analysis of where the time is currently going. As a new faculty, this may not be helpful because you may not know what all your tasks are, and it is understood that a novice at any task needs longer to master his or her work. So what is most effective for new faculty to manage important roles in their lives? Planning, particularly planning in "units of semesters," is most effective.

Think of the calendar year in three units: August to December, January to May, and June/July. If your college uses a different academic semester or you have a 12-month contract, adjust your units accordingly. Consider the following suggestions to organize your academic life.

1. Decide where you will do your class preparation, home office or college office. Leave all your books in one place. Some college offices are prone to having books "walk," so consider the safety of your professional library.

2. Set up an organization system. Decide if lecture (or problem-based) topics will be in notebooks, file folders, computer presentations, or on index cards. Think long term because over your academic career, you may teach 20 different occupational therapy classes. I use manila file folders for each lecture or lab topic. I file all folders in hanging files, clustered by course, in short two-drawer filing cabinets. Each file drawer holds about three courses. I use the filing cabinets to hold up a long kitchen counter top, creating an especially long desk. The desktop holds my computer and several wood crates that form bookcases.

Reprinted from Sladyk, K. (2001). *Clinician to Educator: What Experts Know in Occupational Therapy.* Thorofare, NJ: SLACK Incorporated.

TABLE 13-1

FACULTY, STUDENT, AND CLINICIAN STRESS LEVELS OVER TIME

	Last 3 Weeks of Aug	First 3 Weeks of Sept	Early Oct	Midterm Week	Week After Midterm	Late Oct to Mid Nov	Mid Nov	Late Dec to Dec	Early Jan
Faculty	10	4	7	4	9	9	10	6	2
Students	1	4	6	9	6	7	9	1	1
Clinician	6	6	6	6	6	6	6	6	6

1=relaxed, 5=typical work stress, 10=extreme stress

3. Think about your needs for other roles. As occupational therapists, we are concerned with a person's varied roles, yet as educators, we often neglect our own roles during busy periods. Because each of us is different with different responsibilities, only personal reflection can address this area. In my case, I am prone to frequent interruptions and am involved in diverse causes and projects. If you have children, end of April to early May might be especially busy with dance recitals, award banquets, or scout projects. Avoid heavy correcting assignments in busy times in other roles.

4. Think about the material things that simplify your life. Plan to have enough of these supplies to last weeks. Consider paper plates and cups for busy times. Walk around your home and make a list titled, "Things That Ease My Mind." Buy these items in bulk. For example, I have favorite brands of shampoo, tissues, and paper towels. Each July, I buy in bulk to last me months. I repeat the process in January.

5. Organize your clothing. It may sound silly, but there will be times when laundry will pile up because you are busy reading 55 orthopedic treatment plans. Have enough underclothes to last a long time. Buy clothes that are interchangeable in your favorite color family and do not need special cleaning. Buy socks in limited colors and all the same so you do not have to sort them out of the dryer. Consider laundry service by the pound when things get really busy.

6. Buy stamps and gifts in bulk. Buy a roll of 100 first class stamps and at least ten $3.50 priority stamps. Pick up the free priority envelopes and boxes at your local post office when you buy the stamps. If you send gifts to distant friends and family or give gifts locally, pre-buy phone cards, gas cards, fast food gift certificates, or department store cards for easy mailing and no wrapping later in the semester. Pre-address 6 months' birthday cards or orthodontist payments. If you send Christmas cards, buy, stamp, and address them in October or early November because after Thanksgiving, your workload tends to increase.

7. Refill your medicine cabinet. The college campus is an exciting community that unfortunately spreads cold and flu like wildfire. Each July and January, check your supply of over-the-counter medicines to face a firewall of possible symptoms. As a faculty, there will be days when you need to meet your classroom responsibilities, and you will need some symptom relief to do so. Buy cold, cough, sore throat, and flu supplies enough to cover you and your family for an extended time. Consider a small over-the-counter stash of supplies for the office.

8. Think about your taxes and your retirement. As a professor, you have unique opportunities for tax write-offs that were not available to you as a clinician, but you need to plan ahead because April 15th is a busy time in the academic world as well as the tax world. Specific books on tax issues are available for professors, or consult your tax advisor in July, not April. Further, most colleges or universities use TIAA-CREF for retirement management. This organization has specific retirement options only available to professors. Planning a solid retirement now means you will not be correcting papers at age 70.

9. Avoid time wasters. Mackenzie (1997) identifies the 20 time wasters in business, and several have an impact in academia. These include management by crisis, inadequate planning, drop-in visitors/telephone interruptions, personal disorganization, procrastination, and inability to say no. If we were our own client, we could whip out Uniform Terminology and address these issues. If any of these are issues for you, make a plan. But remember, first-year educators have a lot to do in the early years, change is hard, so don't run out and buy a super-mega-giant day planner unless you like that kind of thing.

REFERENCES

Mackenzie, A. (1997). *The time trap*. New York: American Management Association.

Collecting Articles to Read Later

Karen Sladyk, PhD, OTR, FAOTA

I keep each lecture topic in a file folder and group all file folders together in the filing cabinet by course. As I find articles that would enhance a topic, I make one copy and put it in a pile to be read later. Once a month or so, I sort the articles into the file topics. From time to time, the pile gets too big and becomes overwhelming. When this happens, I give myself permission to toss some out. It is impossible to stay cutting edge on every topic, and I remind myself that I'm a facilitator, not the all-knowing expert.

When a Teacher-Focused Syllabus Becomes a Student-Focused Syllabus

Karen Sladyk, PhD, OTR, FAOTA

Literature on student learning clearly advocates for a syllabus to be student-focused, that is, designed with the student's learning needs and clearly designed to support student development. A teacher-focused syllabus is often viewed as incomplete and old fashioned. The problem with a student-focused syllabus is that it sometimes increases the teacher's workload.

I am advocating for a new definition of teacher-focused syllabus that makes both the teacher and students happy while still allowing the syllabus to be student-centered. Begin by designing an ideal class outline. What would you do if everyone wanted to be in your class and no one was involved in other life roles that could interfere with learning? Evaluate what is reasonable work, considering the credit load and the overall philosophy of the department.

Knowing that students appreciate and need timely feedback, look at the class outline and your personal schedule for the next semester. Having an assignment due after a long holiday weekend may initially be preferred by the students, but if the educator does all correcting on weekends and the following weekend is open house, students may become upset that the assignment will not be returned for 2 weeks. Guilt and pressure may lead the educator to stay up too late correcting an assignment he or she would rather read differently. Now tension, real or imagined, is set up between the educator and the students.

A teacher-focused syllabus designed around a feasible correcting schedule will make students happier in the long run. The teacher should look at his or her personal and professional schedule when assigning due dates to projects. Are there family plans for a wedding the same weekend a term paper/treatment plan is due? Is the term paper due the last week of class when the registrar needs grades 24 hours after the last class? Does a large treatment plan paper really meet the outcome objectives of the class, or can an assignment that is easier to correct meet the objectives better? Are papers or projects due in every class the teacher has at the same time? Can papers be cosigned by two class peers before the teacher reads it, so grammar and technical errors are less likely to slow the reader down? Can practical exams be videotaped and viewed at a more leisurely schedule instead of the teacher sitting there for every session?

One effective way to arrange a more flexible correcting schedule is to have assignments due to the educator's office on a date and time the class does not meet. Most assignments do not need an exact week to complete. Assignments for a Wednesday class may be due by noon on Monday to the teacher's office to allow the teacher to correct during his or her free time on Tuesday. To reduce missing papers, always have assignments due to the office and do not accept assignments in a different class or in the hallway.

Connecting with the Right People on Campus

Karen Sladyk, PhD, OTR, FAOTA

Although you will likely meet and get to know many other faculty and academic administers, forming a relationship with the people of housekeeping, maintenance, the bookstore, media services, and food services will often further your successful academic career.

How Much Is Your Time Worth?

Karen Sladyk, PhD, OTR, FAOTA

Because academic professionals often have numerous projects active at the same time, they are often juggling many balls at once. This is usually manageable until a surprise activity interferes. Sometimes, even simple tasks like mowing the lawn, grocery shopping, or mopping the floors can send a busy schedule over the edge and increase the anxiety of the semester to the boiling point.

My sister taught me a valuable lesson on managing these "crisis" times. Estimate the monetary value of your time. If you were working (conference, per diem, consulting), what would your take-home pay be after taxes? Generally, occupational therapy professors could estimate this from $30 to $65. Cut that in half to an estimated $15. If you can pay anyone else $15 or less per hour to do some work for you, hire them. If you have children yourself, neighborhood or church teens, a stay-at-home mom nearby, or a retired handyman available and interested in odd jobs, hire that person. In my household, the children have family responsibilities in chores that are not paid, but there is a list of available jobs posted when someone is looking for extra cash. In addition, I sometimes pay their friends if they are looking for extra work. I also use a handyman service and laundry by-the-pound service in town.

Reprinted from Sladyk, K. (2001). *Clinician to Educator: What Experts Know in Occupational Therapy.* Thorofare, NJ: SLACK Incorporated.

Chapter Fourteen

RESOURCES FOR FACULTY SUPPORT

Karen Sladyk, PhD, OTR, FAOTA

The following annotated bibliography is provided as resources for new faculty teaching occupational therapy. Other database searches will find more numerous listings, but this is a good place to start when looking for initial support. The listing includes resources from adult education and occupational therapy sources.

Baez, B., & Centra, J. (1995). *Tenure, promotion, and reappointment: Legal and administrative implications.* San Francisco: Jossey-Bass. (Discusses problems and due process in employment contracts and peer review.)

Beer, V. (2000). *The web learning fieldbook.* San Francisco: Jossey-Bass. (Create effective learning environments on the web.)

Berk, R. A. (1998). *Professors are from Mars, students are from Snickers.* Madison, WI: Mendota Press. (A humorous view on why students and teachers see things differently.)

Bligh, D. (2000). *What's the use of lectures?* San Francisco: Jossey-Bass. (Reviews the benefits and abuse of lectures.)

Bonwell, C., & Eison, J. (1991). *Active learning.* San Francisco: Jossey-Bass. (Create excitement in the classroom.)

Brayley, C. R. (1996). *From clinician to academician: A handbook for those who aspire to become faculty members.* Bethesda, MD: American Occupational Therapy Association. (A handbook specifically designed for occupational therapy.)

Brookfield, S. (1991). *Developing critical thinkers.* San Francisco: Jossey-Bass. (Challenging adults to explore alternative ways of thinking and acting.)

Caffarella, R. (1994). *Planning programs for adult learners.* San Francisco: Jossey-Bass. (Theoretical and practical guide for those planning adult education programs.)

Chaffee, J. (1998). *The thinker's way.* Boston: Little, Brown and Co. (An eight-step program to creative thinking.)

Crist, P. (Ed.). (1999). *Innovations in occupational therapy education 1999.* Bethesda, MD: American Occupational Therapy Association. (Numerous articles on a variety of educational issues for occupational therapy.)

Crist, P. (Ed.). (2000). *Innovations in occupational therapy education 2000.* Bethesda, MD: American Occupational Therapy Association. (Numerous articles on a variety of educational issues for occupational therapy.)

Cross, P., & Steadman, M. (1996). *Classroom research: Implementing the scholarship of teaching.* San Francisco: Jossey-Bass. (Design simple research projects for teachers and students.)

Domince, P. (2000). *Learning from our lives.* San Francisco: Jossey-Bass. (Using experience to reinforce learning in adults.)

Evers, F., Rush, J., & Berdrow, I. (1998). *The bases of competence: Skills for lifelong learning and employability.* San Francisco: Jossey-Bass. (Create practical and valued learning experiences for adults.)

Hayes, E., & Flannery, D. (2000). *Women as learners.* San Francisco: Jossey-Bass. (Analyzes learning from a woman's perspective.)

Jarvis, P. (1998). *The practitioner-researcher.* San Francisco: Jossey-Bass. (Learning by doing education bridging theory and practice.)

Jones, D., & Watson, B. (1990). *High risk students in higher education.* San Francisco: Jossey-Bass. (Examines minority, female, low-income, and disabled student factors.)

Menges, R. (1999). *Faculty in new jobs: A guide to settling in, becoming established, and building institutional support.* San Francisco: Jossey-Bass. (Helpful inside information to novice teachers.)

Murray, J. (1995). *Successful faculty development and evaluation: The complete teaching portfolio.* San Francisco: Jossey-Bass. (Use of the teaching portfolio to improve teaching and college culture.)

Nolinske, T. (Ed.). (1999). Special issue on faculty development. *American Journal of Occupational Therapy, 53*(1). (Fifteen articles related to teaching occupational therapy.)

Shapiro, N., & Levine, J. (1999). *Creating communities of learning.* San Francisco: Jossey-Bass. (A basic guide to learning community development.)

Stage, F., Muller, P., Kinzie, J., & Simmons, A. (1998). *Creating learning centered classrooms.* San Francisco: Jossey-Bass. (Reviews research and theory on college learning.)

Stanton, T., Giles, D., & Cruz, N. (1999). *Service learning.* San Francisco: Jossey-Bass. (Pioneers of service learning reflect on its practice.)

Sugar, S. (1998). *Games that teach.* San Francisco: Jossey-Bass. (Crowd-pleasing activities that are educational.)

Ukens, L. (2000). *Energize your audience.* San Francisco: Jossey-Bass. (Seventy-five activities to get them going.)